Collin Gow, C.N.C.

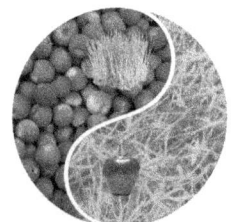

Collected Works on Health and Nutrition, Volume 1 (2017-2020)

Collin Gow, C.N.C.

Contents

Intro

Collin Gow, C.N.C.'s Healing Principles

1. **First do no harm** (The Hippocratic Oath, "First do no harm", should always be a practitioner's #1 priority.)
2. **Eat foods/medicines that are as close to nature as possible** (Forage for wild edibles, but be extremely careful in doing so. Never eat something you are not 100% sure you have identified as edible and never eat more than a very very small amount the first time eating it. Eat wild, fresh off the tree/bush, raw (if edible and healthy in raw form) foods and/or grow your own food. Eating 51% of your foods raw is a good goal.)
3. **Eat whole foods** (Avoid isolates, highly processed, and highly refined foods. See #10.)
4. **Eat a variety of foods** (Biodiversity (variety) is what ensures balance, health, and survival in nature and you *are* nature. Plus, nearly every country in the world recommends getting a variety of foods in your diet as part of their food guidelines.)
5. **Observe and study non-human animals** (Non-human animals know more about health and nutrition than you do, because they are closer to nature than you are. Learn from them. Eat seasonally, drink water that has minerals in it, don't overly sanitize foods, chimpanzees eat high fruit, even herbivores eat small amounts of animal foods.)
6. **Mimic other long living countries' diets** (Drink lots of matcha like in Japan, eat lots of dark chocolate like in Switzerland, eat lots of fermented foods like in South Korea. These people live longer than Americans.)
7. **Mimic traditional cultures** (Mimic their methods of food preparation such as slow, wet heat cooking instead of fast, dry heat cooking. Eat the whole animal including the organs, not just the muscle meat. Soak, sprout, ferment. Mimic their priorities of simplicity, community, family, rest, environmental friendliness, etc.)
8. **Your recent ancestors were hunter-foragers** (Learn from them. They ate high fiber, high omega 3, high fruit and veg, high variety, and omnivorously. They soaked, sprouted, and fermented. They woke up when the sun rose, slept when the sun set, moved naturally, wore natural clothing, got outside, had a tribe, went barefoot, were thankful, and learned survival skills.)
9. **Addition, not subtraction** (Add foods to your diet rather than subtracting too many of them from your diet. Subtracting too many foods leads to a narrow diet, which leads to nutritional deficiencies.)
10. **Everything in nature and every food in nature is both good AND bad** (Nothing is purely good or purely bad, all foods are both good and bad; one should weigh the good against the bad and decide for oneself whether the good outweighs the bad.)
11. **Antidotes, not subtraction** (Animals consume antidotes such as clay to neutralize "toxins" in foods rather than cutting those foods out of their diets and rather than refining out the unpleasant parts of foods. Take a lectin blocking supplement and drink clay, these will neutralize some of the "toxins" in foods and allow you to keep a variety of foods in your diet and avoid deficiencies.)

12. **Find a balance between eating to live long and eating to feel good** (Eating to live long, you may not feel well. Eating to feel well, you may not live long. Find the balance.)

13. **Personalize your diet** (There is no "best" diet. The best diet is *your* diet that *you* figure out through study and trial and error on your own body. Your body is different than everyone else. Know thyself. Know your blood type, genotype, ancestry, metabolic type, dosha, natal chart, conditions, lifestyle, etc.)

14. **180** (Just as Gaia, Earth herself sees fit to reverse her poles 180 degrees every few thousand years to bring balance to herself, just as cells depolarize in response to certain stimuli, so you should reverse and do a 180 on what you eat every now and then to find balance. The weakness of many diets is that they want you to stick to them! Variety is one of the most important principles in my approach. However, I do not exclude the importance of the reverse or the opposite principle from time to time, to bring balance to your diet. I believe in the unity of opposites, lokahi, taijitu, yin within yang and yang within yin, complementary opposites. So, a diet based on variety would not be as wise or as complete if it did not include it's opposite. A narrow diet is the opposite of a diet containing lots of variety. A narrow diet can be useful and beneficial temporarily sometimes, it's just not a good long-term idea. Go 180 every now and then, however. Go narrow every now and then. For example: eat nothing but fruits and veggies for 3 days or eat nothing for a day. These experiments in restriction rather than variety could be a good way to detox, give your body a rest, rebuild your potassium stores, be reminded of the value and power of fruits and vegetables, or could be a good way to remind you of the value of variety. Every experiment is a learning experience. 180 is a principle that embodies the necessity to experiment every now and then as well as a way to continue to progress in your self and dietary awareness through the unity of opposites.)

15. **Overall health, not just labeled diseases and conditions** (See the forest in the trees. Treat not only specific, labeled diseases and conditions you may have, but foster overall health as well.)

16. **Healing crisis** (Be willing to feel worse before you get better. Be willing to put up with minor symptoms like gas, or detox reactions such as a headache, or Herxheimer reactions like a rash or others, in order to get greater gains. That being said, not everything is a healing crisis. Go to the emergency room if you are really concerned.)

17. **Cures are a myth** (A cure, in the sense that something can permanently get rid of or fix a disease or condition, is illusory, it's not real, it doesn't exist, there's no such thing. Let's say a doctor "cures" your cancer. Ok, does that guarantee that it won't come back, if you go back to the same diet and lifestyle habits that caused it? No. Cures are daily maintenance. You must make healthy choices every day to stay healthy and "cured". You must manage your issues. You are deluding yourself if you think some magic remedy is going to fix you once and for all, for all time.

18. **Therapeutic dose** (Usually, you need to triple, quadruple, quintuple, and sometimes even sextuple what the bottle says to achieve a therapeutic dose. What the bottle says is fine for maintenance, but usually you need more than what the bottle says to really address a specific ailment. However, be sure to talk to an experienced practitioner before doing so. This principle is not true of some supplements. Some supplements, such as non-whole-food b-vitamins, are usually way over-formulated, and you actually need less than what the bottle recommends.)

19. **Power of synergy** (There are appropriate occasions for simplicity and appropriate occasions for complexity or synergy. Buying a formula that contains multiple remedies, however, will usually be better for you and work better than one remedy alone. There are no single remedies in Chinese medicine, for instance. They know that formulas with multiple remedies in them are more balanced, wiser, and more effective than single remedies. In a Chinese medicine formula there's a Chief or Principal herb, a Deputy or Minister herb, an Assistant herb, and an Envoy or Courier or Guide herb. Each play a specific role in the formula to balance it properly. From an experimental standpoint, however, sometimes it's good to go simple so you know what is doing what.)

20. **Assistant herbs** (As I mentioned above, Chinese medicine formulas have "Assistant" medicines in them. The role of the Assistant is to counteract and offset the side effects or toxicities of the Chief and the Deputy herbs as well as to augment and strengthen their function. This principle is similar to principle #11, only it's applied to herbal formulas, whereas #11 is applied to foods.)

21. **One layer before another** (You may need to fix some other ancillary layer of your malady/maladies before you can fix the main malady.)

22. **Patience, it's a process** (Rome wasn't built in a day. When you go natural, you may need to make many changes to get healthier that aren't going to happen overnight. Give it time. You may need to tweak things in your regimen multiple times before you get it right. Health is an art, not a science.)

23. **Anything that is not natural is poisonous** (You are a natural animal, you are not a synthetic robot. Anything that is synthetic, or against nature, is by definition poisonous. Pharmaceutical drugs and vaccines are poisonous because they are synthetic. All synthetic products are poisonous.)

24. **No such thing as "side effects" only effects** (The pharmaceutical industry has tricked people into thinking there is such a thing as a side effect. There is no such thing. There are only effects.)

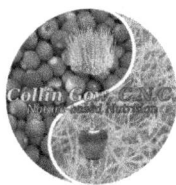

Lifestyle

1. **Read** (It makes you feel smart. We all like to feel smart and knowledge is power.)

2. **Journal** (great way to reflect, clarify your thoughts, de-stress, and keep you on track towards goals)

3. **Breathe deeply** (A longer inhale, and shorter exhale can assist in activating the parasympathetic nervous system and may reduce stress.)

4. **Find your meditation** (Find whatever activity quiets your mind and do it more often, such as tai chi, yoga, stretching, meditating, prayer, getting a massage, taking a bath, taking a walk in nature, doing art, talking with a friend, etc.)

5. **Do what you love** (Make time for what you truly love to do rather than letting life pull you in too many directions away from your true passions. You'll be happier and more inspired.)

6. **Exercise when you can** (you'll feel better about yourself afterward and rid yourself of pent up tension)

7. **Try new and meaningful experiences** (Take a class on something you think you might enjoy, travel to somewhere you've never been to, this expands your social circle, sphere of influence, keeps you learning, and keeps life fresh and interesting.)

8. **Get outside into nature!** (Sunshine increases vitamin D, elevates mood, blue and green colors in nature are relaxing, going barefoot grounds us, reduces oxidative stress, and makes us feel like a kid again!)

9. **Community** (Socializing with your friends and family and participating in a community or tribe is important. Those who are isolated and lonely don't live as long as those with a more active social life. No, social media doesn't count!)

10. **Sleep** (at least 8 hours a night - without rest, there can be no recuperation or healing)

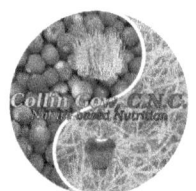

Articles

Eating Organic Versus Conventional Foods

By Collin Gow, C.N.C.

What are the differences between organic foods and conventional foods? Which should you buy? What does it mean to eat organically? Opinions vary so let's gain a basic understanding of the topic. Organic foods are grown and raised with more natural farming methods and food processing techniques, including more natural herbicides, pesticides, fungicides, fertilizers, and animal living conditions, etc. There are strict regulations on organic foods and products, with the National Organic Standards Board, The National Organic Program, and the USDA setting the standards.

From USDA.gov:

"USDA certified organic foods are grown and processed according to federal guidelines addressing, among many factors, soil quality, animal raising practices, pest and weed control, and use of additives. Organic producers rely on natural substances and physical, mechanical, or biologically based farming methods to the fullest extent possible."

The substances below are generally prohibited in organic products:

Genetically modified organisms (GMOs)
Synthetic substances
Nonagricultural substances
Ionizing radiation
Sewage sludge
Antibiotics
Hormones
Artificial preservatives, colors, and flavors

Some natural substances that are toxic are prohibited as well, such as strychnine and arsenic. However, some synthetic substances are allowed, such as pheromones and vaccines. In addition, in order to be labeled organic, no prohibited substances may be applied on the soil within the past 3 years. Processed, organic foods are allowed to contain some approved, non-agricultural ingredients like enzymes, pectin, or baking soda. "Made with organic", processed, multi-ingredient products are their own category with their own stipulations. They must contain at least 70% organic ingredients and cannot bear the USDA organic seal. In regard to animals, it is required that they are raised in accordance with more natural living conditions. For instance, they must be fed 100% organic feed and forage and be allowed natural behaviors, like grazing on pasture.

Concerns over the pricing of organic foods and skepticism over their benefits have led some consumers in the past to not purchase organic products. However, I contend that eating organic is healthier for people, animals, and the planet. Synthetic chemicals pollute water ways and the environment at large. Synthetic pesticides have been shown to be neurotoxic[1] and endocrine disruptors[2]. Eating organically versus conventionally has been shown to reduce urinary pesticide excretion, meaning, eating organic foods reduces the amount of pesticides in one's diet and body[3]. However, according to the researchers referenced that found this, there is insufficient evidence to show relevant and meaningful health outcomes. According to another study called the NutriNet-Santé Prospective Cohort study, published in the Journal of the American Medical Association - Internal Medicine, "high organic food scores were inversely associated with the overall risk of cancer". This means that eating organic food was associated with a reduced risk of cancer[4]. However, other studies have not shown clear benefits. Lastly, a systematic review on organic versus conventional food consumption published in the journal Nutrients stated, "Significant positive outcomes were seen in longitudinal studies where increased organic intake was associated with reduced incidence of infertility, birth defects, allergic sensitisation, otitis media, pre-eclampsia, metabolic syndrome, high BMI, and non-Hodgkin lymphoma."[5] As far as pricing of organic goes, perhaps it is best to think about whether one prefers to pay now or maybe end up paying a doctor's bill later. If one wishes to save money in the short term however, eating more fruits and vegetables and less animal products may help, as healthy produce is almost always cheaper than healthy animal foods. In addition, one can just choose to only buy organic foods if they are on the "dirty dozen" list and buy the rest of their food needs from conventional sources. If it were me, though, I would buy all organic whenever possible.

The Dirty Dozen
(These foods are generally higher in herbicides and pesticides):

Strawberries
Spinach
Kale
Nectarines
Apples
Grapes
Peaches
Cherries
Pears
Tomatoes
Celery
Potatoes

Besides the possible health benefits shown in research, and other than the health advantages that my family and I have seen from eating organic, I have also found that organic food tastes much better too! And world-renowned chefs generally choose to cook with organic foods for that very reason. Plus, food is supposed to be organic folks. That's how nature created it. Think about it. All food was naturally organic prior to WWII and the invention and deployment of synthetic chemical pesticides. Organic food *is* food. Conventional, GMO foods can get so scary that their seeds are actually registered as pesticides, not as food, as in the case of GMO corn seeds. And do you really want spider genes in your goat milk? Fish genes in your tomatoes? Bacterial genes in your corn? GMO pigs that glow in the dark due to jellyfish genes? Atlantic salmon with genes from Pacific salmon and ocean pout? This is frankenfood. Would you want these "foods" in your body? In the environment? Anyway, GMOs are a complex subject for another article. So, for now, I'll leave it at that. The bottom line is, in my opinion, organic food is better, and we shouldn't be labeling organic foods as organic, as if they are the exception. We should instead be labeling foods as conventional. They should be the exception, everything else should be organic and not need a label!

With the number of positives, and clear ways to save money, I say, why not choose organic? As a certified nutritional consultant, I hope that you will choose organic too and reap the rewards as I have.

References:

1 Jett, DA; Neurotoxic pesticides and neurologic effects. Neurologic Clinics 2011 Aug;29(3):667-77.

2 Mnif, Wissem et al. "Effect of endocrine disruptor pesticides: a review." International journal of environmental research and public health vol. 8,6 (2011): 2265-303. doi:10.3390/ijerph8062265

3 Vigar, V.; Myers, S.; Oliver, C.; Arellano, J.; Robinson, S.; Leifert, C. A Systematic Review of Organic Versus Conventional Food Consumption: Is There a Measurable Benefit on Human Health? Nutrients 2020, 12, 7.

4 Baudry, Julia et al. "Association of Frequency of Organic Food Consumption With Cancer Risk: Findings From the NutriNet-Santé Prospective Cohort Study." JAMA internal medicine vol. 178,12 (2018): 1597-1606. doi:10.1001/jamainternmed.2018.4357

5 Vigar, V.; Myers, S.; Oliver, C.; Arellano, J.; Robinson, S.; Leifert, C. A Systematic Review of Organic Versus Conventional Food Consumption: Is There a Measurable Benefit on Human Health? Nutrients 2020, 12, 7.

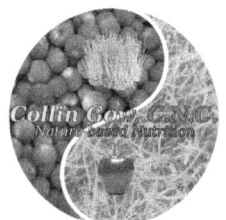

"Postbiotics"
Collin Gow, C.N.C.

Recent research has shown that **not all the benefits of probiotics come from them being alive**. In 2002, 4 different non-living fractions of a particular strain of probiotic bacteria, *Bifidobacterium Bifidum*, had significant immunoregulatory effects. Fractions and extracts from *Bifidobacterium* and *lactobacillus* spp. have also demonstrated strong *in vitro* (in a petri dish) anti-tumor effects. There is much more research than just these studies, however, but first, let me explain.

There are two main terms in the medical literature that comprise the potential gains of either **dead probiotics** or of **byproducts** produced from living probiotics or secreted after cell lysis (cell wall rupture). The first word is "paraprobiotics". Paraprobiotics are "non-viable probiotics", "inactivated probiotics", or "ghost probiotics", basically dead probiotics, which may confer host benefits. The other more phonetically pleasing word, dubbed "**postbiotics**", also known as "metabiotics", "biogenics", "metabolites", or "cell-free supernatants", consist of soluble factors/products or metabolic byproducts secreted by live probiotics or products released after bacterial lysis (cell lysates) which offer physiological benefits. These "bacteria-derived factors" may include **enzymes, peptides, teichoic acids, peptidoglycan-derived muropeptides, endo- and exo-polysaccharides, cell surface proteins, short chain fatty acids, vitamins, plasmalogens, and organic acids**. For convenience sake, I am going to refer to paraprobiotics and postbiotics both as postbiotics. Advantages of postbiotics are a **longer shelf-life** than probiotics, a **clear chemical structure**, and their **safety**. Some harmful effects have been shown from some types of probiotics in certain people, which I'll discuss later on, making postbiotics a safer alternative. Postbiotics are also easier to control, being that they are not live bacteria with the ability to replicate at different rates. Does all this mean that you shouldn't worry about whether the bacteria in the probiotic supplement you buy are dead or alive because either way you are getting a benefit? Not necessarily. Most probiotics are removed from their original growth medium and freeze dried, then put into a capsule. If those probiotics die within an hour of you consuming them, or many of them are already dead, well you'll get some benefit, but not as much as if you ate a fermented food such as kefir and the probiotics died in your gut within an hour. The fermented food would retain all the "postbiotics", some of which are removed when bacteria is stripped of its food growth medium and put into a capsule. There are a few probiotic capsules on the market that keep the original culture medium, and therefore all the postbiotics intact, but very few. You can get positive effects regardless of which way you go, but **not as much postbiotic effects from a regular probiotic capsule as a food**. On to more research.

Efficacy

Postbiotics **possess immunomodulatory, anti-inflammatory, hypocholesterolemic (cholesterol lowering), anti-obesogenic (fat burning), anti-hypertensive (blood pressure lowering), anti-proliferative (anti-cancer spreading), and antioxidant effects**. Anti-inflammatories IL-8, IL-10, and IL-12 have increased in studies on postbiotics. A postbiotic of an *L. paracasei* strain of bacteria protected healthy tissue from *Salmonella* in another study. An *L. casei* strain was able to **mitigate inflammation** in post-infectious bowel syndrome patients. An *L. rhamnosus* GG postbiotic **protected colonic smooth muscle cells** against lipopolysaccharide damage. Lipopolysaccharides are endotoxins found in the outer membranes of bad bacteria. Postbiotics of many different *L. plantarum* strains have **inhibited multiple pathogenic bacteria**, such as *E. coli*, *Salmonella*, and *Enterococci* (which is antibiotic-resistant). One particular postbiotic – lipoteichoic acid has a good variety of benefits. Postbiotic short chain fatty acids are beneficial for lipid metabolism, insulin sensitivity, cholesterol balance, glucose balance, and metabolic balance. Postbiotics from multiple bacterial species of particular strains of probiotics such as *L. fermentum*, *Enterococcus lactis*, and *L. acidophilus* **protect the liver** from toxicity. Postbiotics from *Saccharomyces boulardii* (a yeast often recommended for diarrhea) improved **wound healing** in one study.

Postbiotics may be beneficial for animals as well. Multiple studies have shown that post-biotics may **enhance growth performance in animals** such as hens, broilers, and piglets. Maybe we should be using these bacteria derived factors instead of feeding animals corn and grain or injecting them with hormones to try to get them to grow faster and bigger. Or in addition to zinc and iron, we could use them for children who are not growing at the proper rate.

Safety

Caution needs to be exercised when taking live bacteria (probiotics) just like anything you put in your mouth. **Not all studies on probiotics show benefit, and others show harm**. Yet, the sentiment in the health food industry is that probiotics are all good for you and there seems to be little concern over their potential harm. Caution should especially be exercised in immuno-compromised patients and patients with acute inflammation. One clinical study found that 16% of people with acute pancreatitis given a mixture of probiotics died versus only 6% in the placebo group. In another study, a particular strain of the probiotic *Lactobacillus plantarum* **caused inflammation** similar to *Salmonella* in healthy and non-healthy Irritable Bowel Disease tissue ex vivo. Other *Lactobacillus* strains caused no inflammation in healthy tissue but showed the potential to cause harm in non-healthy IBD tissue. This led the researchers to conclude that **probiotics may be better for patients in remission rather than the acute phase of disease**.

Probiotics may eat the lining of your gut also, especially in the absence of fiber. Bacteremia (bacteria in the blood) is a potential problem as well. Some are suggesting links between probiotic supplements and Small Intestinal Bacterial Overgrowth (SIBO) nowadays also. Lastly, harmful effects such as microbial translocation (microbes breaching the gut wall and translocating into other areas of the body), horizontal gene transfer (when genes transfer from one species of bacteria to another) of antibiotic resistant genes to harmful microorganisms, infection, increased inflammation response, and other problems have been shown with some types of probiotics, more commonly probably soil-based organisms than lacto and bifido bacteria, and more commonly probably in people with compromised immune systems. **Postbiotics possess fewer** of these **risks** as they do not contain live bacteria. While this all may sound frightening, the majority of studies on probiotics show that they are safe and beneficial. And to put this in perspective, **any prescription drug that you take will most likely have exponentially more harmful side effects than a little old probiotic supplement**. Yet, obviously, postbiotics are more appropriate than probiotics for patients with significant risk factors. If you do not have significant risk factors, such as being in an acute phase of a disease, then the best way would probably be to get it all. Take a probiotic supplement from time to time (preferably higher in *Bifidobacteria* than *Lactobacilli*), eat probiotic rich foods containing more postbiotics, and get plenty of prebiotic fiber in your diet or in supplement form.

Secondary metabolites of soil bacteria, or soil-based postbiotics if you will, **play key roles in soil ecology**. These metabolites are involved in cell-cell communication between microorganisms and plants ensuring a balanced, healthy soil which translates to healthier crops. Yet, soil-based organisms applied to human health, while many studies have indicated definite benefits to the host, may be a bit riskier than cow derived or human derived *Lactobacilli* and *Bifidobacteria*, as soil-based organisms are able to form spores and biofilms and can be antibiotic resistant. Perhaps this would be the best application of the use of postbiotics rather than probiotics, using postbiotics from soil-based organisms in humans as a safer alternative to humans consuming soil-based probiotics. We could culture the soil-based organisms on food, then remove or destroy the organisms and feed that food with all its postbiotics to humans instead of taking the actual organisms themselves in capsules. Or we could culture them, then extract the postbiotics only and put that in supplement form. Another interesting idea I had was to make homeopathic soil-based organism products. Homeopathic medicine is not fooey. It is a legitimate science as demonstrated by the Germans for years and as proven by Luc Montagnier, the man that discovered the aids virus. Water is able to register and store the vibrations or frequencies of things within its coherent domains. So, we could code the vibration or frequency given off by certain soil-based organisms into water and consume those supplements rather than the bacteria themselves, just a thought.

Anyhow, microbial metabolomics, or the science or study of microbe metabolites and their effects on human cells, is an interesting area involving cutting edge research in the fields of health and nutrition. Probiotics and their postbiotics have already been shown to influence the expression of the human genome in epigenetic fashion. **Postbiotics overall safety and their ability to still favorably alter the human microbiome (the ecosystem of organisms in your gut) despite being absent of live bacteria, or absent of bacteria altogether, make them a great choice for those who are very sensitive to supplements and/or foods and who want to take their gut health journey more slowly.** For more information on postbiotics and how you can get them into your diet or to learn alternative ways to get probiotic benefits without taking live bacteria, contact me at collingowcnc@gmail.com and we can set up a consultation. This has not been an attempt to treat, diagnose, prevent, or cure any disease or condition. As usual, talk to your naturopath before making any changes.

References:

Aguilar-Toalá, J.E., García-Varela, R., García, H.S., Mata-Haro, V., GonzálezCórdova, A.F., Vallejo-Cordoba, B., Hernández-Mendoza, A., Postbiotics: An evolving term within the functional foods field, Trends in Food Science & Technology (2018), doi: 10.1016/j.tifs.2018.03.009.

Besselink MG, van Santvoort HC, Buskens E, et al. Probiotic prophylaxis in predicted severe acute pancreatitis: a randomised, double-blind, placebo-controlled trial. Lancet 2008;371:651–9.

Tsilingiri K, Barbosa T, Penna G, et al Probiotic and postbiotic activity in health and disease: comparison on a novel polarised ex-vivo organ culture model Gut 2012;61:1007-1015.

Mahesh S. Desai et al. A Dietary Fiber-Deprived Gut Microbiota Degrades the Colonic Mucus Barrier and Enhances Pathogen Susceptibility. Cell, November 2016 DOI: 10.1016/j.cell.2016.10.043

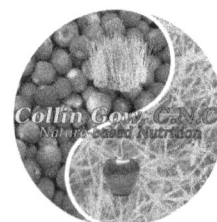

Type-1 Diabetes, Causes and Nutritional Approaches for Blood Sugar Control

by Collin Gow, C.N.C.

Diabetes Mellitus Type-1 affects **1 in 300 people** in the United States according to large epidemiological studies. About 5% of people with diabetes in general have type 1. It is an **autoimmune** disease with many possible causes where the immune system attacks the **beta cells** of the pancreas. This results in either complete destruction of the function of beta cells or partial destruction leading to an **inability to produce sufficient amounts of insulin** and amylin. Without adequate insulin supply, blood sugar remains very high causing **vascular damage, neuropathy, retinopathy, kidney damage, and other complications**. Amylin is a peptide hormone that is co-secreted with insulin from the beta cells which slows gastric emptying and promotes satiety, thereby preventing post-prandial (after meal) glucose spikes. So, not only does one not produce enough insulin to control blood sugar, but one also loses some of the ability to feel full and some of the ability to self-prevent spikes in blood sugar. The majority of cases of type 1 diabetes are diagnosed at a young age, which is why it was once referred to as juvenile diabetes, but it **can be diagnosed at any age**. Symptoms of type 1 diabetes may include:

- Frequent urination
- Excessive thirst
- Increased hunger
- Weight loss
- Blurry vision
- Fatigue
- Poor healing
- Bed wetting
- Irritability

If left untreated, diabetic ketoacidosis may occur, which is a condition of excess, poisonous, acidic **ketones** in the blood that are produced in response to having to utilize fats and proteins for energy instead of glucose. Some of you may have heard of ketogenic diets purported online and in health food stores as a way to lose weight. The goal is to eat no carbohydrates or very very low amounts of carbohydrates in order to burn fat. There is mixed research out there on ketogenic diets for Alzheimer's disease and epilepsy. However, in my opinion, this diet should almost never be done long-term because it is **far too acidic** to remain healthy and if one is avoiding carbohydrates, that means one is avoiding fruit, which may inevitably lead to potassium deficiency. Potassium is required by the body in higher amounts than ANY other mineral. Symptoms of ketoacidosis include:

- Flushed, hot, dry skin
- Rapid, deep breathing
- A strong, fruity breath odor
- Loss of appetite

- Belly pain
- Vomiting
- Confusion

What causes type 1 diabetes?

Many potential causes have been put forward over the years of what causes type 1 diabetes. For the most part, **environmental agents are thought to trigger it in those who are genetically at risk. Nutritional deficiencies also put one at risk.** Here are some of those environmental agents, deficiencies, and genetic risks.

MAP

Also known as *Mycobacterium avium subspecies paratuberculosis*, MAP is a **bacteria** that has been **linked to type 1 diabetes** in multiple studies since 2005. Live MAP bacteria have been found in pasteurized milk, infant formula made from pasteurized milk, beef, pork, chicken, surface water, soil, cow manure, and municipal tap water. MAP is thought to induce type 1 diabetes via a mechanism called **molecular mimicry**. In the case of molecular mimicry and MAP, what happens is the body produces "heat shock proteins" in response to stress caused by the infection of the bacteria. Some of these heat shock proteins **mimic pancreatic glutamic acid decarboxylase**, or **GAD**. The MAP does this in order to hide from the body's immune system. Confusion ensues and the body starts producing antibodies against its own pancreatic tissue. Testing for anti-GAD antibodies is one way to confirm type 1 diabetes. GAD is responsible for the **synthesis of GABA** in the body, an inhibitory neurotransmitter that calms the nervous system and may reduce anxiety. Supplemental GABA may be a specifically important option for people with type 1 diabetes. **The link between GAD, type 1 diabetes, and the particular MAP heat shock protein was established as early as 1990** by a study published in The Lancet, volume 336, No.8715. Disproportionate amounts of MAP have been found in the blood of type 1 diabetics versus healthy controls AND versus type 2 diabetics. Antibodies against MAP bacteria proteins in type 1 diabetics have been found in multiple studies out of Italy and in one study out of Sardinia called the TRIGR study. In fact, **7 out of 8 studies on MAP and type 1 diabetes showed a significant association between the two.** It is interesting to understand why the 8th study did not find a link between MAP bacteria and type 1 diabetes. The 8th study came out of India and some explanations were put forward as to why they did not find an association, such as, possible cross protection from *Mycobacterium avium ssp. paratuberculosis* due to commonplace vaccination for regular tuberculosis, high incidences of vegetarianism, or the compulsory boiling of milk that Indians often do before consuming it. **Boiling may destroy MAP better than pasteurization.** To avoid contracting too much MAP bacteria consider consuming animal foods less often, buy from local dairies with more quality control, or buy raw milk and boil it yourself or take a probiotic with it. Also, after handling raw meat, be sure to wash your hands and arms with hot soapy water for at least 3 minutes and cook your meat until well done. If you absolutely must have your steak bloody or medium temperature, then consuming natural antimicrobials such as berberine at the same time, wouldn't be a bad idea. In fact, whenever primates consume meat, they always consume bitter leaves with it to prevent infection and to aid digestion.

Cow's Milk

Many studies indicate an association between **early exposure** to cow's milk in infants and type 1 diabetes. The TRIGR study mentioned above furthered this research and compared regular cows-milk based infant formula versus **hydrolyzed** cows-milk based infant formula and showed a lower incidence of type 1 diabetes in the hydrolyzed group. However, this is only half the story. Around 2,000 or more years ago a mutation in Northern European cows caused them to produce the protein **casein A-1** in their milk instead of the usual casein A-2. Casein A-1 is more difficult to digest than casein A-2 causing more bloating and upset stomach. However, once it is digested, casein A-1 turns into **a lectin-like** protein called **beta-casomorphin-7**. This protein pries open the gut, enters the blood stream, and attaches to the beta cells of the pancreas, causing the immune system to attack them, another case of mistaken identity. Products like **Restore**, and other leaky gut supportive products may help mitigate breaches of the intestinal wall by lectins, plus, breakdown in tight junction proteins in the kidneys of type 1 diabetics has been shown in studies and Restore may possibly improve tight junction function in the kidneys also. According to a study published in the Nutrition & Diabetes journal in 2017, **"A1 β-casein consumption correlates significantly with type 1 diabetes incidence and shows a stronger correlation than does milk consumption *per se.*"** To ensure you or your children are not consuming casein A-1 at all, either avoid dairy altogether, or choose goat, yak, sheep, camel, buffalo, or donkey dairy products instead of cow dairy products. In addition, you may ask your dairy provider whether their cows are predominantly A-1 producing or predominantly A-2 producing, or whether they are Holstein, Friesian, Ayrshire, and British Shorthorn cows (A-1) or Jersey, Guernsey, Brown Swiss, or Belgian Blues (A-2).

Genetics

A genetic polymorphism in humans on the gene called **SLC11A1** may make a person more at-risk for type 1 diabetes. SLC11A1 activates macrophages that engulf pathogens such as MAP. Therefore, if a person has a mutation on this gene, then they are more susceptible to *Mycobacterium avium paratuberculosis* infections. Also, people with genetic susceptibility to **autoimmune thyroid diseases** often are also genetically susceptible to type 1 diabetes showing an interesting thyroid link to the picture. Supporting the thyroid may be of some help to type 1 diabetics. The most important statement as to the genetic causes of T1D that I have found is this: **"Genes located within the HLA class II region on chromosome 6p21 account for approximately 50% of genetic risk for T1D"** (Wherrett et al., 2009). 23andme.com is one way to get all of your raw genetic data, which may then be plugged into different websites like geneticgenie.org that can interpret some of the data for you.

Vitamin D Deficiency

A meta-analysis published in 2013 in the journal Nutrients stated, "…vitamin D intake during early life may be associated with a reduced risk of type 1 diabetes." A study in 2008 found that incidences of type 1 diabetes were **higher at higher latitudes** with lower UVB radiation (Mohr et al., 2008). Higher latitudes get less sunlight, generally. The less sun, the less vitamin D your body produces. Pregnant mothers may want to consume at least 5,000 IU of vitamin D3 per day to ensure that their levels are high enough and 1,000 IU for infants is a safe and effective level for baby to consume as well. However, talk to your naturopath or holistic pediatrician to see what levels they recommend.

Celiac disease, **enterovirus infections** in childhood, and the **overuse of antibiotics** may trigger the disease as well.

What supplements may be of help for blood sugar control?
Cayenne

Capsaicin, a compound found in cayenne pepper has been shown in studies to possess **insulinotropic** activity in mice with type 1 diabetes, causing increased insulin secretion, yet at the same time it does not cause hyperinsulinemia. In many cases this resulted in a reduction in blood sugar, but not in all cases. Cayenne has been studied for **neuropathy** as well, a common complication of diabetes, showing lower pain scores in many cases. Many clients and customers over the years have reported to me good results with their blood sugar levels in response to taking cayenne supplements. In addition, peppers are some of the highest food sources of vitamin C. If you are suffering from rheumatoid arthritis, however, because peppers are in the **nightshade** family, you may want to limit their intake.

Gymnema

One of the best options for sugar control may be a potently bitter herb called *Gymnema Sylvestre,* also known as **"sugar destroyer"**. Gymnema possesses multiple mechanisms of action on blood sugar and has been studied in mice with type 1 diabetes and in humans with type 2 diabetes. A review published in 2015 in the Evidence Based Complimentary and Alternative Medicine Journal pinpointed some of these effects. Gymnema may increase insulin secretion, decrease plasma glucose levels, and **regenerate pancreatic beta cells**. Gymnema also has the potential to **block excess sugar absorption** and if you let it sit on your tongue for a few minutes before swallowing, it can inhibit your taste buds from tasting sweets. Plus, with use in Ayurvedic medicine for thousands of years, it has history on its side.

Berberine

Berberine is a bitter **alkaloid** contained in herbs such as goldenseal, barberry, Oregon grape root, and others. It is commonly used to treat diabetes and diarrhea in China. Berberine increases insulin in a dose-dependent manner, meaning, normal concentrations increase pancreatic insulin secretion, while extremely high concentrations actually decrease pancreatic insulin secretion. A study in the Journal of Biological Chemistry, 2009, reported that **berberine prevented the progression of type 1 diabetes in 50% of the mice studied after just 2 weeks**. Berberine also reduced inflammation in the study. Other studies on berberine show an increase in insulin sensitivity in type 2 diabetic mice. It has also been shown to **attenuate intestinal barrier damage** in type 2 diabetic mice. I always refer to berberine as the next curcumin. The amount of research I have seen on berberine and the variety of issues it may help is staggering and, at the right dose, I think it deserves to be in the spotlight of almost anyone's regimen for overall health.

Bitter Melon

We are beginning to see a clear theme here about what may help to keep your blood sugar within a healthy range. **Bitters**. The bitter taste is the taste you ought to be looking for in your foods if you wish to control your blood sugar and increase insulin production. In China, bitter melon is eaten as a vegetable and has been referred to as **"vegetable insulin"**, though, botanically speaking, it's actually a fruit. It contains a protein called polypeptide-p, or, **p-insulin**, which is structurally similar to human insulin. "The p-insulin works by mimicking the action of human insulin in the body and thus may be used as plant-based insulin replacement in patients with type-1 diabetes" (Joseph et al.), Asian Pacific Journal of Tropical Disease, 2013. Treatment with a water extract of bitter melon **prevented apoptosis (cell suicide) in pancreatic beta cells** in *vitro* (in a petri dish) as reported by a study published in 2007 in the Asia Pacific Journal of Clinical Nutrition. The Molecular Cell Biochemistry journal published a study in 2004 showing a significant **increase in pancreatic beta cell numbers in rats** receiving daily oral administration of bitter melon juice compared to untreated diabetic rats. One should be careful of consuming bitter melon seeds, however, as the vicine content may have good as well as bad effects on the body. Supplement manufacturers are usually aware of this.

Many other nutraceuticals and therapies that show potential benefits for blood sugar balance in type 1 diabetics in the medical literature exist, such as, **vanadium and pregnenolone (may help regenerate beta cells), niacinamide, rosemary, biofeedback assisted relaxation, omega 3 fatty acids, vitamin E, and more**. For blood sugar regulation in general, **b-vitamins, chromium, cinnamon, green coffee bean, and apple cider vinegar** are strong choices as well. Of course, sticking to an organic, anti-inflammatory, low glycemic, high fiber diet may also be important for regulating blood sugar. Pick low sugar fruits such as blueberries, kiwis, green apples, and greenish bananas, coconut products such as shredded coconut or coconut butter, high omega-3 foods such as chia seeds, walnuts, and wild caught salmon, and controlled portions of buckwheat, quinoa, and semi-cooked sweet potatoes with beans and dulse are good choices. Beans slow the digestion of carbohydrates, helping reduce blood sugar spikes, while seaweeds like dulse may help to block the lectins in beans that have been associated with digestive upset. Probiotic-rich fermented foods are important, as studies show a decline in the amount of and the diversity of good gut bacteria preceding the onset of type 1 diabetes. Of course, leafy greens are fair game, the more you eat, the bitter, I mean better. As a caveat, **be sure to talk to your Dr. before undergoing any changes to your diet or adding any new supplements to your regimen.** I hope this article added a few pieces to the puzzle of type 1 diabetes, increased your knowledge on the subject, and may be of assistance in the management of your blood sugar.

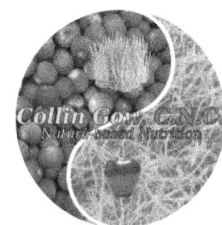

Serrapeptase

Amazing Enzyme Studied for Pain, Stiffness, Inflammation, Sinusitis, Arthritis, and More!

For the millions of people who take anti-inflammatory medications to relieve pain and promote cardiovascular health, there is a supplement that shows amazing promise. The name of this supplement is Serratiopeptidase, commonly known as Serrapeptase, and doctors in Europe and Asia have been prescribing it to treat everything from pain to atherosclerotic plaques for nearly 40 years. It is similar to other anti-inflammatory enzymes such as **pancreatin, bromelain, papain, nattokinase, lumbrokinase, streptokinase, urokinase, trypsin, and chymotrypsin**. However, during the 1980s and 1990s it was proposed by separate research conducted in Europe and Japan that Serrapeptase was the most effective agent in reducing inflammation among all other enzyme preparations. Some say Lumbrokinase is the strongest, but it depends on what you are going for and I have not been able to confirm this through research, plus it is harder to come by at health food stores, so Serrapeptase is usually the best option.

Serrapeptase is a **proteolytic, fibrinolytic,** and **caseinolytic** enzyme that is produced by culturing the enterobacterium *Serratia* sp. E-15. This bacterium was originally discovered and isolated from the intestines of silkworms, which synthesize it in order to break down the walls of their cocoons after undergoing transformation into a moth. No need to wormy, I mean worry, however, because silk worms have not been involved in the culturing process since it was isolated from them in the 60s. In humans, this enzyme mainly helps to reduce inflammation and improve circulation by lysing or breaking up something called **fibrin** – a tough, stiff, fibrous, cross-linked, **insoluble protein** produced by the action of **thrombin** on **fibrinogen**, which causes blood clots, cysts, and blocks circulation. The build-up of this stiff, thready protein can contribute to making your body stiff, thready, tight, and tense. Wouldn't you rather be strong, flexible, and relaxed? Joint tissue is already avascular, meaning it has no direct blood flow to it. The effect of lysing this damaged, non-functional, dead protein fibrin cannot be understated, as many people with chronic pain conditions lack adequate circulation, after all, cardiovascular disease is the number one killer in America. There are many potential causes of high levels of fibrinogen (and therefore fibrin) in the body, such as deficiencies of particular nutrients including **omega 3s, vitamin C, silica, vitamin k2, lysine, proline, glycine, and b-vitamins,** as well as other possible causes such as **viruses, bacterial infections, heavy metals, intestinal permeability, low testosterone,** and certain **genetic defects** to name a few. So, taking some of these nutrients or addressing some of the other possible causes may provide other alternative long term approaches for fibrinogen maintenance besides taking Serrapeptase (more on this subject later). However, Serrapeptase is proving to bring rapid relief for those uncertain as to the causes of their high fibrinogen levels and it is quickly becoming a possible alternative to NSAIDs (Non-Steroidal Anti-Inflammatory Drugs) often used to treat rheumatoid arthritis and osteoarthritis. Serrapeptase has been used by doctors to treat many conditions including chronic sinusitis, carpal tunnel syndrome, sprains and torn ligaments, fibrocystic breast disease, ovarian cysts, ear, nose and throat infections, fibromyalgia, varicose veins, emphysema, asthma, bronchitis, migraines (vascular), Inflammatory Bowel Diseases (IBD) including Crohn's, colitis and cystitis, enlarged prostate, pain, and postoperative inflammation. Some researchers believe Serrapeptase can play an important role in arterial plaque prevention and removal as well.

NSAIDs are commonly used to treat pain, inflammation, rheumatoid arthritis and osteoarthritis. Nonselective (COX1 and COX2) NSAIDs include Ibuprofen, Acetaminophen, and salicylates (Aspirin). With the numerous reports linking NSAIDs and other COX2 enzyme inhibiting drugs to heart attacks, stroke, intestinal bleeding, kidney or liver impairment, many are looking for safe, natural alternatives. Opioids used to treat chronic pain with their side effects such as sleepiness and potential for addiction and anti-depressants prescribed for pain with their increased risks of suicide and libido killing effects are not great options either. According to data released in 2012 by the Alliance for Natural Health International, the risk of death from pharmaceutical drugs in the UK is **62,000 times** higher than the risk from taking food supplements. Also, unlike over-the-counter NSAIDs, Serrapeptase has not been shown to cause ulcers or stomach bleeding.

Inflammation:

A clinical trial published in the Journal of Pharmacology and Pharmacotherapeutics compared the anti-inflammatory activity of Serrapeptase and Diclofenac (NSAID) in rats and discovered an almost equivalent effect, with Serrapeptase **reducing inflammation 68%** and Diclofenac **72%**. Serrapeptase was also demonstrated to **reduce histamine** in the study. Our bodies have a love-hate relationship with inflammation. On the one hand, inflammation is a natural response necessary to protect the body from invading organisms and is necessary for repairing tissues. On the other hand, excessive, or chronic inflammation can limit joint function, and destroy bone, cartilage and other joint structures. Serrapeptase may be of help for excessive inflammation by **thinning and draining the fluids** formed from injuries. Another clinical trial out of the Indian Journal of Pharmaceutical Sciences in 2008 studied the effect of proteolytic enzymes and aspirin on **swelling** (edema) induced by inflammation in rats and found a **62.81% reduction** with Serrapeptase, beating out trypsin, chymotrypsin, and aspirin. One of the other ways Serrapeptase reduces inflammation is by **dissolving fibrin**, as I have mentioned. Reduced fibrinolysis, and therefore high fibrin levels, was associated with rheumatoid arthritis in the journal *Nature* in 2012. In addition, one study out of the Journal of Immunology in 1995 showed that fibrin induces the expression of the pro-inflammatory cytokine **IL-1 beta** which in excessive amounts has been implicated in hair loss, wrinkles, and the **degeneration of cartilage and collagen**. Another study out of the same journal of the same year showed that fibrin induced **leukocyte chemotactic factor** and **IL-8** in vivo. Crohn's disease sufferers generally have high IL-8 levels. This suggests that Serrapeptase, with its **potent fibrinolytic activity** may be of use for some important kinds of inflammation.

Pain Reduction:

While Serrapeptase reduces inflammation, one of its most profound benefits is reduction of pain, due to its ability to block the release of pain-inducing amines such as **bradykinin** from inflamed tissues. Lumbrokinase also performs this feat. Bradykinin **raises intracellular calcium levels** and causes the **release of glutamate** which may over-excite the nervous system creating more **pain** and the potential for **cell death**. Lowering bradykinin levels may **calm the nervous system** and **protect cells**. The beneficial circulatory effect may assist with pain management as well. Researchers showed that patients with long-term lower back pain had **constricted blood flow**, and those with high cholesterol appeared to suffer with more severe symptoms. Those with narrowed arteries appear about **8.5 times** more likely to have suffered from chronic back pain than those without narrowed arteries. So, Serrapeptase with its **clot dissolving** action may be of some help. The best-selling joint pain supplement in the health food industry is **Terry Naturally Curamin**, which contains only 4 ingredients and one of those ingredients is a proteolytic enzyme. It has won 28 awards since its creation. Obviously these enzymes are assisting very well with pain relief.

Post Operative Swelling and Pain:

In Germany and other European countries, Serrapeptase is a common treatment for inflammatory and traumatic swellings. One double-blind study was conducted by German researchers to determine the effect of Serrapeptase on post-operative swelling and pain. This study involved **66 patients** who were treated surgically for fresh rupture of the lateral collateral ligament of the knee. On the third post-operative day, the group receiving Serrapeptase exhibited a **50% reduction of swelling**, compared to the controls. The patients receiving Serrapeptase also became pain-free more rapidly than the controls, and by the tenth day, the pain had disappeared completely. A study of **24 healthy individuals** with impacted molars in 2008 out of the International Journal of Oral Maxillofacial Surgery showed a significant **reduction in swelling and pain intensity** after molar surgery.

Fibro-Cystic Breast Disease/Scar Tissue/Fibromyalgia:

Serrapeptase has been used in the successful treatment of fibrocystic breast disease. In a double-blind study of **70 women** published in the Singapore Medical Journal in 1999, Serrapeptase was found to be superior to placebo for improvement of breast pain, breast swelling, and induration (firmness). **85.7%** of the patients receiving Serrapeptase reported moderate to marked improvement. No adverse reactions to Serrapeptase were reported. Researchers concluded that Serrapeptase is a safe and effective method for the treatment of breast engorgement. This evidence points to possibilities for the use of Serrapeptase on other kinds of cysts such as those occurring on the ovaries in polycystic ovarian syndrome. There is anecdotal evidence of the use of Serrapeptase for dissolving scar tissue also, as scar tissue is another kind of non-living fibrous tissue containing high levels of fibrin. I gave Serrapeptase to a woman with constipation due to a bowel blockage caused by scar tissue that had formed post bowel surgery and within 1 week it was gone. Further, the word FIBROmyalgia would seem to be another likely candidate for some help from the use of Serrapeptase. There is a condition of hypoxia (low oxygen) in the muscle and joint tissue of fibromyalgia patients, so the circulatory benefit of Serrapeptase could likely **increase oxygen** to these areas.

Alzheimer's and Dementia:

Amyloid fibrils and cross linking are involved in the progression of Alzheimer's disease. Some proteolytic enzymes have been studied to **degrade** and **reduce amyloid fibrils** and **increase oxygen** to the brain and many have been studied to **decrease cross-linking** of damaged proteins. You may know cross-linking by another name: advanced glycation end products. These **AGES** age your cells drastically, cause inflammation, and have been implicated in the progression of cataracts, nephropathy, and many other conditions.

Sinusitis:

Due to its anti-inflammatory properties, Serrapeptase has been shown in clinical studies to benefit chronic sinusitis sufferers. In this condition, the mucus in patients' nasal cavities is thickened and hyper-secreted. This thickening causes mucus to be expelled less frequently. Japanese researchers evaluated the effects of Serrapeptase (30 mg/day orally for four weeks) on the elasticity and viscosity of the nasal mucus in adults with chronic sinusitis. Serrapeptase **reduced** the **viscosity of the mucus**, improving the **elimination of bronchopulmonary secretions**.

Ear, Nose and Throat:

Other clinical trials support Serrapeptase's ability to relieve the problems associated with ear, nose, and throat infection, anosmia (loss of smell), nasal obstruction, laryngitis, difficulty in swallowing, often in just 3-4 days. Physicians assessed efficacy of treatment as excellent or good for **97.3%** of patients treated with Serrapeptase compared with only **21.9%** of those treated with a placebo. One anecdotal report indicated that Serrapeptase ended years of snoring literally overnight.

Biofilms:

Biofilms are sticky conglomerations of protein, fibrin, heavy metals, DNA, lipids, cells, and polysaccharides produced by some harmful pathogens to protect themselves from your own immune defenses. Some of these pathogens include *Candida Albicans* and the genus *Borrelia,* which causes Lyme disease. Dissolving biofilms can be a necessary part of **penetrating and killing harmful pathogens** as well as **detoxifying heavy metals** from the body. Proteolytic enzymes like Serrapeptase have the ability to help **digest** the **cell walls and biofilms** of some of these pathogens. One **study** conducted by Italian researchers suggests that proteolytic enzymes could significantly **enhance the activities of** the **antibiotics** ofloxacin, ampicillin, ciclacillin, cephalexin, minocycline, and cefotiam against biofilms.

Carpal Tunnel Syndrome:

A small study of **20 people** out of Sawai ManSingh Medical College and Hospital in India studied the effects of carpal tunnel syndrome over the course of **6 weeks**. Participants took 10mg of Serrapeptase twice daily. At the end of the study, **65%** of the participants showed **significant improvement**. No significant side effects were observed.

Cardiovascular Health:

Cardiovascular implications and the **fibrinolytic, clot dissolving** effect has been shown by Hans A. Nieper, M.D., an internist from Hannover, Germany, where he studied the effects of Serrapeptase on plaque accumulations in the arteries. The formation of plaque involves deposits of fatty substances, cholesterol, cellular waste products, immune cells, calcium and fibrin on the inner lining of the arteries due to inflammation. Excessive plaque results in partial or complete blockage of the blood's flow through an artery, resulting in arteriosclerosis, and potentially a stroke or heart attack. The evidence to support Serrapeptase's role in preventing plaque build-up is anecdotal. Still, further studies are called for in this area as Nieper's research indicated that the protein-dissolving action of Serrapeptase will gradually **break down atherosclerotic plaques**.

According to Dr. Nieper, 30,000 I.U. of Serrapetase per day for 12 to 18 months is sufficient to remove fibrous blockages from constricted coronary arteries, as confirmed in many of his patients by ultrasound examination. As a certified nutritional consultant, I will recommend, on an empty stomach, anywhere from **40,000 SPUs** once per day, up to **120,000 SPUs** two to three times per day, depending on the person and their specific health challenges. I have had many people report their success stories to me after recommending Serrapeptase, which I will be happy to share with anyone interested. One customer told me just the other day, "Hey, I just have to tell you: that is the best supplement I have ever taken!" "I took 1 before bed and when I woke up in the morning I could actually breathe for the first time in years." Not everyone taking it will have the same extraordinary results, but for many, it may prove to be the missing link they have been looking for.

Before getting your hopes up too much, there are a few important things to know before taking Serrapeptase. Many of the studies on Serrapeptase are for **short term use**. Fibrin and plaque, while contributing to clots and strokes, do play an important role in protecting your blood vessels from rupture. Taking high doses of Serrapeptase long term and stripping too much plaque and fibrin out of your body without providing the proper raw materials to create new healthy tissue to replace the plaque and without doing things to strengthen the blood vessels, some issues may come up, as you would be losing the protective role of the plaque. One case of pneumonia infection was linked to Serrapeptase as reported by a hospital in Japan. The 84-year-old patient had been taking Serrapeptase for chronic cystitis for 3 months as prescribed by his doctor. Therefore, I like to recommend **silica, lysine, proline, glycine, glycosaminoglycans** and either **pine bark, rutin, or grapeseed extract** in conjunction with it for the safest long term use of the supplement and for the best effect. Eating more greens or taking **vitamin K1** may also be appropriate. Otherwise, I recommend cycling on and off of Serrapeptase periodically, or try **nattokinase** as a milder option for more long term use. Also, if you are taking a blood thinner, you may want to consult your holistic physician before taking it. And remember, Serrapeptase and other proteolytic enzymes should be taken on an **empty stomach** to work properly. In addition, products like **Dr. Chi's Vein Lite, Oxypower,** and **Joint Force** may be of help for joint pain, circulation, and inflammation and may produce similar effects to Serrapeptase, or try adding **MSM, boswellia, buffered vitamin C,** and **hemp oil** to your circulation and anti-inflammatory regimen for more support. If you are looking for more results for stiffness, tightness, tension, or muscle pain, then **magnesium, MSM,** and **apple cider vinegar** are great go to's. Apple cider vinegar and **iodine** may help with proteolysis due to their ability to raise body temperature and due to their low ph. **Garlic, turmeric, royal jelly,** *lactobacillus acidophilus, lactobacillus plantarum*, **exercise**, and **frequent consumption of nuts and seeds** have also shown to **lower fibrinogen levels** in studies. Research out of Australia in 2007 showed that *lactobacillus casei* **L26 and** *lactobacillus delbrueckii ssp. Bulgaricus* **Lb 1466** had the highest proteolytic activity among 8 probiotic strains studied. *Bacillus subtilis* is a soil-based probiotic that is responsible for the production of the fibrinolytic enzyme nattokinase. The Hadza consume a heavily plant-based diet, contributing to a microbiome enriched in unclassified members of **Bacteroidetes** and **Clostridiales**, which are groups of bacteria known for their fibrinolytic capabilities. Lastly, **Enterococcus faecalis** TH10 is a probiotic strain considered by some to possess strong proteolytic activity.

In conclusion, studies have shown that if you suffer from inflammatory diseases, rheumatoid arthritis, osteoarthritis, sinusitis, carpal tunnel syndrome, snoring, fibrocystic breast disease, ovarian cysts, fibromyalgia, varicose veins, Inflammatory Bowel Disease, migraine headaches, enlarged prostate, tennis elbow, lung problems, arteriosclerosis, edema (swelling), pain, or cardiovascular plaque build-up, then Serrapeptase, in combination with a healthy diet, may provide the relief you've been searching for without the side effects of NSAIDs and other drugs. It is important to have a balance of proteolysis in the body, so talk to your naturopathic doctor before making any changes. This article is not an attempt to treat, diagnose, prevent, or cure any disease or condition, simply a survey of a fraction of the research on this fascinating supplement.

Thanks to the tiny larvae of the silk moth, researchers have taken a giant leap toward finding relief for inflammatory disease sufferers.

References:

MR aortography and serum cholesterol levels in patients with long-term nonspecific lower back pain. Spine (Phila Pa 1976). 2004 Oct 1;29(19):2147-52.

Prevalence of stenotic changes in arteries supplying the lumbar spine. A postmortem angiographic study on 140 subjects. Ann Rheum Dis. 1997 Oct;56(10):591-5.

http://www.journal-surgery.net/article/S1743-9191(13)00026-5/abstract

Fibrinogen as a key regulator of inflammation in disease. Semin Immunopathol. 2012 Jan;34(1):43-62. doi: 10.1007/s00281-011-0290-8. Epub 2011 Oct 31.

Proteolytic Enzymes: a New Treatment Strategy for Prosthetic Infections? 12ANTIMICROBIAL AGENTS AND CHEMOTHERAPY, Dec. 1993, p. 2618-2621

Study of garlic effect on fibrinolytic activity of the blood clot in vitro. *Iranian Journal of Pediatric Hematology Oncology Vol1.No2.*

http://umm.edu/health/medical/altmed/herb/turmeric

Nut and Seed Consumption and Inflammatory Markers in the Multi-Ethnic Study of Atherosclerosis. Am J Epidemiol (2006) 163 (3): 222-231. DOI: https://doi.org/10.1093/aje/kwj033

https://www.researchgate.net/publication/255973753_Testosterone_and_acute_stress_are_associated_with_fibrinogen_and_von_Willebrand_factor_in_African_men_The_SABPA_study

https://www.researchgate.net/publication/21701603_Changes_in_blood_lipids_and_fibrinogen_with_a_note_on_safety_in_a_long_term_study_on_the_effects_of_n-3_fatty_acids_in_subjects_receiving_fish_oil_supplements_and_followed_for_seven_years

http://ajcn.nutrition.org/content/76/6/1249.full

http://www.sciencedirect.com/science/article/pii/S1214021X1630206X

http://www.sciencedirect.com/science/article/pii/S0014299908005724

http://www.nature.com/nrrheum/journal/v8/n12/full/nrrheum.2012.184.html

Kee WH, Tan SL, Lee V, Salmon YM. The treatment of breast engorement with Serrapeptase (Danzen): a randomised double-blind controlled trial. Singapore Med J. 1989 Feb;30(1):48-54.

Mazzone A, Catalani M, Costanzo M, Drusian A, Mandoli A, Russo S, Guarini E, Vesperini G. Evaluation of Serratia peptidase in acute or chronic inflammation of otorhinolaryngology pathology: a multicentre, double-blind, randomized trial versus placebo. J Int Med Res. 1990 Sep-Oct;18(5):379-88.

Kakinuma A, Moriya N, Kawahara K, Sugino H. Repression of fibrinolysis in scalded rats by administration of Serratia protease. Biochem Pharmacol. 1982 Sep 15;31(18):2861-6.

Esch PM, Gerngross H, Fabian A. [Reduction of postoperative swelling. Objective measurement of swelling of the upper ankle joint in treatment with serrapeptase– a prospective study]. Fortschr Med. 1989 Feb 10;107(4):67-8, 71-2. German.

Antibiotic susceptibility tests showed that serratiopeptidase (Serrapeptase) greatly enhances the activity of the antibiotic, ofloxacin, and that it can inhibit biofilm formation. [Antimicrob Agents Chemother. 1993; 37(12): pp.2618-21]

https://www.ncbi.nlm.nih.gov/pubmed/11019569

https://www.ncbi.nlm.nih.gov/pubmed/7836771

https://www.ncbi.nlm.nih.gov/pubmed/7608564

https://www.ncbi.nlm.nih.gov/pmc/articles/PMC2852049/

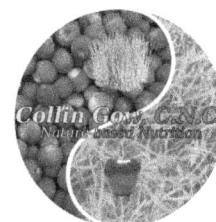

The Chimpanzee Diet

As Homo sapiens, we share 98.5 - 99.4% of our DNA with bonobos and chimpanzees and we are biologically classified in the Order primates, along with macaques, tarsiers, lemurs, baboons, gibbons, gorillas, and orangutans. In addition, gorillas, orangutans, bonobos, chimpanzees, and humans all share all these classifications: Kingdom: Animalia, Phylum: Chordata, Class: Mammalia, Order: Primates, Suborder: Haplorhini, Infraorder: Simiiformes, Family: Hominidae. Some have even debated that chimpanzees should be classified in the same genus as humans, *Homo*, because we only diverged from them 4 to 6 million years ago. Were they classified in such a way, it could improve the rights and person-hood status of chimps and change the way they, and humans alike, are perceived. While we are called "wise man", (*Homo sapiens*) and chimps are not, nevertheless, they are intelligent. They have been observed to use many tools. They use specialized dipping sticks to extract ants and termites from tree hollows and nests, sticks to fish for algae, leaves as sponges or spoons to drink water from, stones or bigger sticks as hammers and exposed tree roots or rocks as anvils to crack nuts, scooping sticks to harvest honey from hives, fluid dipping tools, and other tools. Each of these tools are usually selected and crafted differently for the different purposes. Chimps, among other animals, also display self-medicative behaviors, called zoopharmacognosy. They have been known to consume soil as an anti-malarial, elm bark for bacterial infections, cordia flower stems reducing their risk for tuberculosis, and unripe figs as a de-wormer. They also swallow rough, sand-paper like *Aspilia* leaves or fig leaves and chew the pith of *Vernonia* plants to sweep out and/or kill parasites. The average lifespan of a chimp is 40 - 45 years. Lifespan is not everything, however. It has been argued that many animals, though they may carry many diseases, do not necessarily suffer from those diseases too much because their diets are so medicinal and their self-medication is so natural to them, intuitive, and ingrained into their DNA, daily diet, and way of life. Nearly everything an animal and hunter-forager for that matter eats is medicinal. It is only modern American humans that need to add medicines as adjuncts to their diets and they only tend to do this when they get sick, rather than consuming medicinal foods daily in a preventive fashion. Humans suffer from chronic diseases of civilization that are often absent in other species. What good is a long life, if it is one of suffering? Of course, one could argue that animals suffer in many other ways that humans don't, but vice versa too! But I digress, and that is a big subject for another essay. For the reasons listed above - having similar DNA to chimps, being biologically classified in the same Order as them, seeing that they are intelligent, and appreciating their medicinal know how that eliminates some of their suffering, among other reasons - it would probably be truly wise of us to step down from our speciesist high horse for a moment and compare our current, narrow, deficient, modern American human diets to theirs, our closest-living, almost human, animal relatives, and find out if we can learn something from that comparison.

Common chimpanzees (*Pan troglodytes*) are frugivore-omnivores and have been known to eat a wide variety of foods including figs, other fruits such as African grapes, custard apples, *Mimusops*, and *Musanga* fruits, leaves, flowers, algae, seeds, nuts such as palm nuts, panda nuts, and kola nuts, pith from stems, gums, resins, gum-resins, bark, insects such as beetle grubs, ants, and termites, honey, birds, bird's eggs, crabs, underground storage organs (roots, tubers, bulbs), small mammals, mammals such as blue duikers (small antelopes), bushbucks (another type of antelope), colobus monkeys, red-tailed monkeys, yellow baboons, galagos, aka bush babies, and warthogs. Fruit makes up the majority of their diets and figs are the most popular and available. Specialist wasps pollinate figs and lay their eggs inside. When a fig is pollinated by a wasp it dies inside. Chimps, therefore, sometimes consume figs containing wasp mummies, wasp eggs, or wasp larvae. What about hydration? What do they drink?

They get their fluids from fruit, pools, rivers, tree holes, fermented palm sap, and other sources. Below are some studies showing the percentages of food groups in chimps' diets.

Feeding times of chimpanzees (Pan troglodytes schweinfurthii) at Ngogo, Kibale National Park, Uganda:[1]
191 different plant foods
Mesocarp from non-fig fruits 42.3%
Figs 28.4%
Leaves and leaf buds 19.6%
Seeds 3.95%
Flowers 2.46%
Pith and stems 2.2%
Cambium 0.6%
Roots 0.4%
Other food types 0.1%

Chimpanzee feeding ecology in the Congo Basin (values vary at different times of the year): [2]
158 plant foods plus 18 non-plant foods
92% plants, 8% other
Fruit 55 – 68%
Leaves 2.6 – 16 - 20-28%
Flowers 8%

Feeding behavior of released chimpanzees in Conkouati-Douli National Park, Republic of Congo:[3]
86 plant taxa from at least 42 plant families
Fruits 58%
Leaves 18%
Stem 16%
Seeds 3%
Insects, soil, and meat <3%

Foraging profiles of chimpanzees in the Lopé Reserve, Gabon:[4]
142 species eaten
Fruit 67.6%
Young leaves 9.9%
Mature leaves 1.4%
Immature seeds 2.8%
Ripe Seeds 4.2%
Pith 2.1%
Bark .7%
Flowers 2.1%
Miscellaneous 1.4%
Insects 5.6%
Mammals 2.1%

Some of the aspects that really separate chimpanzees' and other animals' diets from the modern

American human diet (M.A.H.D.), is the variety of foods in their diets versus ours, the diversity and quantity of microorganisms in them, being that they don't usually wash or cook their food, the abundance of minerals they get from drinking unfiltered water and eating dirt, the extra enzymes consumed because their foods are all raw and uncooked, the ubiquitous medicinal foods, and the very astute, self-medicative prowess they have. One of the reasons chimps are able to eat raw meat is that they always consume bitter leaves with the raw meat which helps digest it and helps to kill pathogens. Plus, they usually eat their meat freshly killed. It hasn't been shipped out and sitting in a butcher shop or grocery store for weeks. Chimpanzees obviously must get more vitamin C, antioxidants, and potassium in their diets than us as well from the ample fruit they ingest. Their high fruit diet is an important distinction and there is a strong basis upon which to make the claim that humans should be consuming more fruit than we are. The grounds for this assertion are as follows: 97% of the population is deficient in potassium, it is required in higher amounts than any mineral, humans lack the gulonolactone oxidase enzyme to synthesize vitamin C, probably because we became so reliant on fruit in our primate past that we no longer needed to produce it, a study[5] from 2002 showed that, anatomically, modern humans are unspecialized frugivores whom, for the majority of their evolution, ate mostly plant foods, and lastly, meat as a staple for long periods of time was unlikely. Paleolithic hunter-gatherers ate a good amount of animal foods, yes, and they are more connected to nature than we are and eating a better diet than us, yes, and the *Homo sapiens*, hunter-gatherer diet of the recent 2 or 3 million years (minus the past 10,000 or so since agriculture) contributed to encephalization, our intelligence, and who/what we are today, but the paleolithic period is a blip on the historic/prehistorical hominin dietary record. That doesn't mean it should be thrown out. I'm a big fan of many components of hunter-forager diets and lifeways. Lots of considerations should be made before a person chooses their diet, and even once they choose a diet, it should always be evolving.

Anyway, this brief explanation of the chimpanzee diet, a diet you're not used to hearing enough good information about, is only the fare of one specific species of primate. There is so much more to learn from other primates', other wild animals', hunter-foragers', and other peoples' diets. Hopefully this whets your appetite and thirst for more knowledge in these areas and urges you to read more of my future articles/books on these subjects.

References:
1. Watts, David & Potts, Kevin & Lwanga, Jeremiah & Mitani, John. (2012). Diet of chimpanzees (Pan troglodytes schweinfurthii) at Ngogo, Kibale National Park, Uganda, 1. Diet composition and diversity. American journal of primatology. 74. 114-29. 10.1002/ajp.21016.
2. Morgan, David & Sanz, Crickette. (2006). Chimpanzee Feeding Ecology and Comparisons with Sympatric Gorillas in the Goualougo Triangle, Republik of Congo. Feeding Ecology in Apes and Other Primates, 97-122 (2006).
3. Amandine, Renaud & Jamart, Aliette & Goossens, Benoît & Ross, Caroline. (2013). A Longitudinal Study on Feeding Behaviour and Activity Patterns of Released Chimpanzees in Conkouati-Douli National Park, Republic of Congo. Animals. 3. 532-550. 10.3390/ani3020532.
4. Tutin, C.E. & Fernandez, M. & Rogers, M & Williamson, Liz & Mcgrew, William. (1991). Foraging profiles of sympatric lowland gorillas and chimpanzees in the Lope Reserve, Gabon [and Discussion]. Philosophical Transactions of The Royal Society B Biological Sciences. 334. 179-85; discussion 185. 10.1098/rstb.1991.0107.
5. Claude Marcel Hladik, Patrick Pasquet. The human adaptations to meat eating: a reappraisal. Human Evolution, Springer Verlag, 2002, 17, pp.199-206.

Available for download @ collingowcnc.wixsite.com/collingowcnc/articlesandprotocols

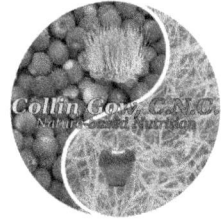

Toxic Vaccine Excipients
and Their Effects

By Collin Gow, C.N.C.

11/24/2020

MRC-5: human fetal lung fibroblast cells originally derived from a 14-week-old male fetus aborted in 1966. In an open letter to legislators regarding fetal cell DNA in vaccines, Dr. Theresa Deisher wrote that human fetal DNA contaminates vaccines and can reach a blood level in a vaccinated child that is known to activate TLR9, which can cause autoimmune attacks. Non-self DNA may cross react with a child's own DNA, according to Deisher. Children with autism have antibodies against human DNA in their circulation and increased levels of autism corresponded to the introduction of and/or increased doses of MMR, varicella, and hepatitis A vaccines containing fetal DNA (Deisher et al.) (https://www.soundchoice.org/open-letter-to-legislators/). Dr. Helen Ratajczak has suggested an increased prevalence of autism from human DNA being added to vaccines too. Also, an increased spike in autism has been documented since the chicken pox virus began being cultured in human fetal tissue for vaccines in 1995 (Ratajczak et al.).

Vero cells: monkey kidney cells which may be contaminated with other pathogenic microbes not intended to be in the vaccine (Osada et al.) (Vilchez et al.).

Human serum albumin: protein from human blood.

Calf bovine serum albumin: protein from the blood of baby cows. A study published in the New England Journal of Medicine found that bovine serum albumin causes membranous nephropathy in early childhood (Debiec et al.).

CRM 197 carrier protein: "non-toxic" mutant of diphtheria toxin, yet some studies have shown it to be toxic to yeast cells and mammalian cells (Kimura et al.). "Functions as a carrier for polysaccharides and haptens, making them immunogenic."

Plasdone C: pyrogen free water-soluble adhesive/polymer.

Anhydrous lactose: water-free milk sugar.

Polacrilin potassium: weakly acidic cation exchange resin/plastic.

Cellulose acetate phthalate: compound consisting of a polysaccharide, often from the cell walls of plants, as well as acetic acid, and an ester of phthalic anhydride. Phthalates are endocrine disrupting plasticizer chemicals banned in some children's toys and banned in cosmetics and personal care products in California and Europe. They may cause rhinitis, eczema, asthma, reduced penile size, incomplete testicular descent, and other issues (Meeker et al.).

Acetone: flammable organic solvent used in nail polish and paint thinner.

FD&C Yellow #6 aluminum lake dye: artificial color shown to cause hypersensitivity reactions (Kobylewski et al.), allergic reactions (EFSA, 2009), attention problems in children (EFSA, 2009), estrogenic activity (Axon et al.), and potentially impact testicular health negatively (EFSA, 2009). Aluminum is neurotoxic (Inan-Eroglu) (Shaw et al.).

Hydrolyzed casein: difficult to digest, allergenic protein from milk linked to type 1 diabetes (Chia et al.). Anaphylaxis reactions to immunizations containing casein have been reported in the medical literature (Silva et al.).

Sucrose: table sugar (a disaccharide containing glucose and fructose).

D-sorbitol: sugar alcohol that occurs naturally but is also produced synthetically and is associated with gastrointestinal disturbances (Mäkinen et al.).

Formaldehyde: one of the most toxic substances known, a carcinogen (Swenberg et al.), corrosive (NJDH 2016), flammable gas (NJDH 2016), used in embalming fluid, is a byproduct of automotive exhaust, and is released from carpet and particle board. It is on the Right To Know Hazardous Substance List as cited by OSHA, ACGIH, DOT, NIOSH, NTP, DEP, IARC, IRIS, NFPA, and the EPA and is also on the Special Health Hazard Substance List. It causes cancer of the nasopharynx and leukemia (NJDH 2016).

Aluminum phosphate/hydroxide: toxic metal shown to cause osteomalacia, microcytic anemia, and encephalopathy/dementia (Willhite et al.). Aluminum is neurotoxic (Inan-Eroglu) (Shaw et al.) and may induce "oxidative stress, immunologic alterations, genotoxicity, pro-inflammatory effect, peptide denaturation or transformation, enzymatic dysfunction, metabolic derangement, amyloidogenesis, membrane perturbation, iron dyshomeostasis, apoptosis, necrosis and dysplasia" (Igbokwe et al.). Aluminum as a vaccine adjuvant can cause autoimmune diseases (Pellegrino et al.) (Dorea et al.) (Perricone et al.), chronic fatigue (Couette et al.), and cognitive dysfunction/deficits (Couette et al.) (Shaw et al.). Aluminum in vaccines can cause macrophagic myofasciitis, muscle weakness, MS symptoms, MS-like demyelinating disorders, etc. (Israeli et al.) (Authier et al.) (Gherardi et al.).

Trometamol: weakly toxic, biologically inert amino alcohol (Spadea et al.), a component of buffer solutions, increases cell membrane permeability. A gel form was associated with periorbital dermatitis (Spadea et al.).

Polysorbate 80 (Tween 80) (polyoxyethylene sorbitan mono-oleate): synthetic nonionic surfactant used widely as an additive in foods, pharmaceutical preparations, and cosmetics as an emulsifier, dispersant, or stabilizer (National Toxicology Program, 1992). Has been associated with an increased risk of systemic adverse events including hypersensitivity systemic reactions (Schwartzberg et al.), a number of reproductive problems in female rats (Gajdová et al.), hypotension and tachycardia in dogs (Millard et al.), and thrombocytopenia, pulmonary deterioration, ascites, and liver and renal failure, secondary to vasculopathic hepatotoxicity in pediatric patients (Kriegel et al.).

Neomycin sulfate: "broad spectrum aminoglycoside antibiotic derived from Streptomyces fradiae with antibacterial activity" (Pubchem). Causes nephrotoxicity and ototoxicity (Masur et al.).

Streptomycin: antibiotic shown to enhance the susceptibility to Salmonella infection (Bohnhoff et al.)

and to enhance Candida growth (Campbell et al.).

Polymyxin B: Antibiotic. Neurotoxic and nephrotoxic (Falagas et al.).

Glutaraldehyde: low molecular weight aldehyde disinfectant. Side effects may include sensory irritant effects, sinus symptoms, and bronchitis (Takigawa), and potential neurotoxicity and developmental effects (Beauchamp et al.). Toxic to fish and birds (Leung et al.).

Host cell DNA benzonase: "genetically engineered endonuclease from Serratia marcescens". "Attacks and degrades all forms of DNA and RNA" (Millipore Sigma). Removes the nucleic acids from recombinant proteins by digesting DNA and RNA. Decreases the viscosity of protein extracts and prevents clumping of chimeric cell mixtures.

Deoxycholate: bile acid. Bile acid does not belong in your blood stream, it belongs in your gallbladder and duodenum.

Octoxynol-10 (TRITON X-100): poly(ethylene glycol) derivative non ionic surfactant. Acts as an emulsifier/detergent to solubilize proteins and permeabilizes living cell membranes (Koley et al.). In excess concentrations, it is fatal to human cells (Koley et al.). Strong evidence that it is a human skin toxicant or allergen (EWG Skin Deep Database).

Ammonium thiocyanate: on the hazardous substance list as cited by DOT and EPA, is a skin, eye, nose, and throat irritant (NJDH 2002), repeated exposure may cause headache, nausea, vomiting, loss of appetite, and weight loss (NJDH 2002), may affect the thyroid gland (NJDH 2002), may cause confusion, dizziness, convulsions, anxiety, and unconsciousness and death (NJDH 2002), harmful to aquatic life with long lasting effects (Labchem 2016), When handling this substance it is recommended to wear gloves, protective clothing, eye protection, and face protection (Fisher Science Education 2014).

Thimerosal: compound containing 49.6% ethyl mercury, a known neurotoxin and cardiotoxin that can cause over 250 symptoms (Dorea et al.) (Azevedo et al.) (Rice et al.). Over 89 peer reviewed articles have linked mercury, thimerosal, and autism (childrenshealthdefense.org). At least 180 studies have shown thimerosal to be harmful (Geier et al.). Six studies done by the CDC showing thimerosal in vaccines to be safe are unreliable and show evidence of scientific malfeasance (Hooker et al.). Boys who received hep B vaccines with mercury were 9 times more likely to become developmentally disabled versus unvaccinated boys (Gallagher et al.)

Live viruses: Many vaccines contain live viruses such as MMR, Varivax (varicella vaccine), Proquad, RotaTeq and Rotarix (rotavirus vaccines), Flu mist, Yellow fever vaccine, Adenovirus vaccine, Chickenpox vaccine, Typhoid vaccine, BCG, Smallpox vaccine, and the Oral Polio Vaccine. Natural measles and mumps infections (as opposed to ones caused by vaccination) in childhood are protective against fatal heart attacks and strokes during adulthood (Kubota et al.). Abnormal MMR antibody levels are found in children with autism and have been linked to MMR vaccination (Singh et al.). Young children are at an increased risk of requiring emergency care after MMR vaccination (Wilson et al.). Vaccinating children against chickenpox increases cases of fatal shingles in the elderly (Brisson et al.) (Luyten et al.) (Ogunjimi et al.). Acquiring chickenpox (varicella) naturally during childhood protects against coronary heart disease (Pesonen et al.) and the universal chickenpox vaccination program is not effective (Goldman et al.). The rotavirus vaccine, RotaTeq, may increase the risk of life-threatening intestinal damage and Kawasaki disease (Geier et al.). Polio vaccination in India probably caused thousands of children to be paralyzed (Vashisht et al.). Millions of people in the U.S. in the 1950's received a polio vaccine that was contaminated with the cancer-causing SV40 virus due to being cultured in monkey kidneys (Shah et al.).

For more information:
https://www.cdc.gov/vaccines/pubs/pinkbook/downloads/appendices/b/excipient-table-2.pdf
http://www.vaccinesafety.edu/components-Excipients.htm
collingowcnc.wixsite.com/collingowcnc/articlesandprotocols

The statements herein have not been evaluated by the FDA. This is not an attempt to treat, diagnose, prevent, or cure any disease or condition. Talk to your doctor before making any changes.

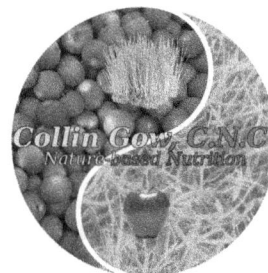

Do Respirators, Surgical Masks, Or Face Coverings Protect Against COVID-19?: Taking the Science and Question in Context

Collin Gow, C.N.C.

June 18, 2020

This article presents information on the pros and cons of wearing face masks and asks the question whether or not they should be part of a healthy approach by the **public** to protecting themselves from COVID-19. **While some of the studies presented within this article talk about masks in medical settings, this article does not address the subject of mask-wearing in medical settings by medical professionals to a large degree, rather it focuses on mask wearing by the public.** I must also preface this article by saying that whether or not one wears a mask is a personal choice. Each person's situation is different and each person should decide for themselves whether or not wearing a mask is the right choice for them and their beliefs about the world. If one chooses to wear or not wear a mask to protect themselves, that's their prerogative. If one chooses to wear or not wear a mask to protect others that's their prerogative. If one chooses to wear or not wear a mask to protect themselves and others that's their prerogative. If one chooses to wear or not wear a mask for social comfort or for other reasons that's their prerogative. **You are responsible for your own health and your own decisions.** I am not liable for what you choose to do. I only present information for your consideration. **You should always talk to your doctor/naturopath before making any changes.** It's also important to know that the science and opinions and policies on a given subject constantly change based on new, developing information. Despite the wishful thinking of some folks, **the science is NEVER settled**. There is no such thing as settled, and this article is not to be construed as a final say on the topic of mask-wearing. Moving on.

The **CDC** currently recommends that "**everyone**" over the **age of 2** wear a cloth **face covering** in public unless they have trouble breathing or are unconscious or cannot remove the mask without assistance. This updated recommendation overturns their previous recommendation that only those who are sick or taking care of the sick should wear one. It is not recommended by the CDC to wear a **respirator** or **surgical mask** as those are to be reserved for healthcare workers and first responders. The **WHO** originally advised the public not to wear masks, like the CDC, unless they are sick or caring for the sick, for fear they would use up supplies needed by medical workers and create a "false sense of security" and now they are saying that the general public should wear a mask in public places where physical distancing is difficult to maintain and in settings of high population density. This updated recommendation comes with a caveat that they admit: "At the present time, the widespread use of masks by healthy people in the community setting is not yet supported by high quality or direct scientific evidence and there are potential benefits and harms to consider", (WHO, 2020). **The U.S. surgeon general**, a member of **The Whitehouse Coronavirus Task Force**, originally cautioned against masks for those who are not ill or taking care of the ill but has now urged the public to wear face coverings, lockstep in line with the CDC. A variety of pundits appearing on **mainstream media television** have recommended that the public wear face masks. Many **governors** have been following CDC recommendations and urging the use of masks too. **Our fellow face mask wearing Americans** are shaming others who are not wearing them, making them feel like they're selfish murderers for not wearing one. With such a disproportionate cry of passionate voices on one side of the subject, often, but not always, blindly following and championing the dictums of our leaders and the rhetoric of the mainstream, the establishment, and the status quo, perhaps it is time to level the playing field, show some actual **scientific research** on the topic, show both sides of the divide, and think about the prospect of mask-wearing in a **broader context**, rather than just unquestioningly accepting the chants and bleats of the herd. Gandhi said, "even if you are a minority of one, the truth is the truth". So let's question. Let's find out the truth. (I am not saying that everyone who wears a mask is blindly accepting what they've been told and doing no research for themselves, nor am I shaming people who are wearing masks. I'm only saying that *some* people are blindly accepting and I am only advocating the questioning of the status quo.)

Let's start with the broader context first, then move on to the scientific research on respirators and masks. If the majority of the public and the majority of the people in positions of power in America are either going along with or at least heeding the CDC and WHO's advice, then perhaps we should investigate these agencies a little bit to see if what they are saying is sound and sage advice or not. **Should we trust the CDC or the WHO or the Coronavirus Task Force or the mass media or governors?** The CDC is a U.S. government agency, but let's remember, in America, there is probably no such thing as government, only the illusion of government, as billionaires and corporations likely own our government through their obscene and exorbitant "donations" and lobbying powers. For example, **Bill Gates gave the CDC $1 million in 2003, $30 million in 2013/14 and he is now the 2nd largest contributor of funding to the WHO behind the U.S. government after giving a combined $20 million to groups that included them and the CDC in 2020 to combat COVID-19. He has given the WHO at least $327 million to date. Don't you think that has an effect on these agencies' suggestions?** The WHO is a United Nations agency. The U.N. has an agenda on record called **Agenda 21 aka Agenda 2030** which seeks to control and reduce the population, vaccinate everyone, sterilize people, take away private land, eliminate rights and freedoms, and establish a global government, under the guise of creating a sustainable future for the planet. If you believe that vaccines are healthy and good for you and are capable of saving the world, well, then you just haven't done enough of your own research, haven't studied the history of vaccination, don't know that **sanitation cured polio, not the vaccine,** don't understand the regulations on vaccines or what they actually mean when they say that they are "safe and effective", don't realize that you cannot legally sue a vaccine company for damages to your child from a vaccine, aren't aware that **getting the flu vaccine may increase your risk of getting coronaviruses by 36%,**[1] or maybe you think that **cancer causing viruses such as SV40, cancer causing chemicals such as formaldehyde (given the highest possible hazard rating there is on the EWG website), demyelinating, nervous system destroying metals like mercury and aluminum, fetal diploid cells, monkey kidney cells, bovine calf serum, chicken embryos, coronaviruses from dogs,** and the rest of the slew of toxic compounds they contain are good to inject directly into your blood stream without negative consequences to your health. One read of *Miller's Review of Critical Vaccine Studies* or one watch of any of Gary Null's vaccine documentaries and you will probably be in tears over how horrific vaccines really are. Even if they are good for you, shouldn't you have a choice about what is injected into your own body? Meanwhile, Bill Gates' money has been responsible for injecting these gruesome ingredients into 760 million children around the world and the vaccination mandates are presently being planned in California and New York to take away your choice, under the influence of none other than Bill Gates, along with other players of course. To each their own, again, each person's situation is different. If you decide to get vaccinated that is your prerogative. Again, I am only defending having a choice over the matter. But vaccines are a HUGE subject for another article. Anyway, here's a little more on William. His numerous grants have granted him a huge influence on the policies that the CDC and WHO put forward. These are not the only agencies Bill Gates has under his thumb either. You better believe it, he has slowly but surely monopolized global, public health through various charitable donations and stock options. Let's remember also, Bill Gates became one of the richest men in the world by creating Microsoft Windows, which was made with an operating system **pirated** from Gary Kildall and Xerox, not entirely of his own creation, he was **sued** by the U.S. government in the 90s prior to his release of Microsoft Windows '98, and **Bill Gates is not a doctor, an epidemiologist, or a certified infectious disease researcher**. And let's not forget that **The Bill and Melinda Gates Foundation is a major funding source for the Pirbright Institute, proud owner of U.S. patent number 10,130,701 B2, a patent approved in 2018 on a coronavirus vaccine**. You think the vaccine will really take a year to develop as you were originally told? Think again. Maybe that's just what they wanted you to believe. My guess is that Bill stands to make a lot of bills by telling us that everyone needs to be vaccinated. By the way, he has also called for a national tracking system to be put in place to know who has COVID-19 and who has or hasn't been vaccinated and his money is already working on giving people quantum dot tattoos for this purpose. Plus, Microsoft, in alliance with Accenture, IDEO, Gavi, and the Rockefeller Foundation and supported by the U.N. is working on ID2020, which may seek to use RFID microchip implants to be able to digitally identify everyone and track them. Then in October/November of 2019, Bill's foundation put on a pandemic "exercise" that "simulated" a major coronavirus outbreak one month **prior** to when the actual coronavirus outbreak occurred in December of 2019 called **Event 201**. At this round-table sat representatives from Johnson and Johnson, Johns Hopkins University, **China CDC**, Bill and Melinda Gates Foundation, ANZ Bank Group, UPS Foundation, UN, Former US Deputy National Security Advisor, US CDC, World Bank Group, and NBC Universal. If you watched this event, as I did, you would have seen that companies were basically jockeying for position, persuading, and promoting the need of the private sector to respond to such a pandemic to get their share of the profits from such a "potential" outbreak. You would also notice how the U.S. CDC representative is wearing a military uniform (maybe the man is ex military) and says, "Governments are going to need to be willing to do things that are out of their historical perspective. For the most part it's really a **war footing** that we need to be on". Another participant from Henry Schein says we need to escalate entrepreneurship and have subsidies and tax breaks given to companies from the government so they can make more products and advocates for a "**MARTIAL type plan**". Martial law anyone? A participant from Edelman basically says that social media platforms need to **censor** misinformation and change their position from being technology platforms to broadcasters and that they need to partner with scientific and health communities to "flood the zone" with "accurate" information. A rep of the Monetary Authority of Singapore wonders if governments should step up their efforts on "enforcement actions against fake news". Bye bye net neutrality. Remember, this event was held BEFORE any public knowledge of any actual pandemic. And what happened a few months later after Event 201 when we were in real, full pandemic mode? The dominoes fell exactly like these people planned. I was personally censored a number of times for my truth-telling Facebook posts, and other "in the know" videos continue to disappear from YouTube daily. What's more, in 2010 **Gates bought 500,000 shares of GMO giant Monsanto** valued at $23 million, Gates' father was on the board of Planned Parenthood, which was birthed out of the **American Eugenics Society**, and, recently, Bill Gates stepped down from being on the board of directors for **Berkshire Hathaway**, the owner of Acme Bricks, the company that allegedly delivered loads of bricks to major cities around the country at the height of the George Floyd protests. This last one is off topic, I know, but is it really? Just continuing the Bill Gates onslaught here, sorry. Another fact of the matter is that **all of these agencies/companies/ individuals generally follow the Big Pharma, allopathic, standard of care, conventional, medical model and generally do not acknowledge alternative medicine nor the natural health industry and often go so far as to call**

it's remedies, some of which have hundreds of thousands of studies on them and a 5,000 year track record of use, safety, and efficacy, far longer than any such invention as synthetic pharmaceutical drugs and vaccines, quackery. And maybe Gates and his CDC have good intentions, maybe Gates believes what he is doing is right, maybe he believes he is improving peoples' health and when you improve peoples' health then they choose to have less kids because they know those kids are more likely to survive, thus justifying the depopulation agenda he admits to in numerous interviews and TED talks. If so, if he thinks he is helping people with all of his "philanthropy" and if he isn't intentionally doing evil, well then that's only because he's a civilized, westernized, modernist and technologist, not a naturopath or naturalist. Maybe it's just ignorance on his part. Maybe it's just completely unbeknownst to him that **modern technology does not give health. Nature gives health. Nature *is* health. And health *is* nature. Health only comes from nature. It has always been so, and will always be so. Anything that is unnatural and does not obey nature's laws always has a side effect and negative consequence.** And maybe we do need to reduce population, but vaccination and GMOs and Planned Parenthood's recommendation that fibroid causing, cancer causing birth control is a "safe and easy way to prevent pregnancy" is not the way to go. Maybe it would be better if we just used our resources more wisely and frugally and funded solar and wind power and electric cars and changed monocrop GMO farming to permaculture farming and offered incentives for having less children and improved family planning education or some other wiser, healthier, more natural method. But enough about all of that. I had to unmask some of the parties involved, though, in this masked debate about face masks, to have an honest conversation about it and provide some context for this proceeding. So, on account of the reasons above, **I think the answer as to whether these agencies and individuals can be trusted to provide the right information as regards our health or not, is probably no**. But I am not the doctor here. Once again, legally I must say that you should probably hear out your government and your doctor before making any decisions. But I didn't even get into **Anthony Fauci** or any of the other goons on the tube telling you what to do. A simple viewing of part 1 of the "Plandemic" documentary will suffice for his indictment, that is, if you can find it, since all major search engines have censored and buried it. I'll give you a little teaser though, Fauci is the director of the National Institute of Allergy and Infectious Diseases which, prior to the pandemic gave $7.4 million to the Wuhan Institute of Virology lab in Wuhan, China that was studying coronaviruses in bats and also, **Fauci owns** multiple patents, one of which is **patent number US20030180254A1, a patent on IL-2 therapy, which is the therapy that he, along with Robert Redfield, current director of the CDC, directed AIDS patients receive during that pandemic back in the 80s, allegedly after 2 years of holding up the confirmation of the virus until the patents were pushed through.** Again, I'm not claiming there's some massive, organized conspiracy and that these people and agencies are doing these things with nefarious intentions, it might just be ignorance or power hunger, or in the case of Fauci greed and ignorance, and they might just be caught up in the same modern machine we are all caught up in that we just can't seem to stop or escape from. Alright alright. Sorry. That's enough for now. The rabbit hole is just so deep I couldn't help myself. Now the stage is set to present some real information on respirators and face masks, not opinion and not conjecture nor secondhand hearsay.

Firstly, what are the **differences** between **respirators** and **surgical masks**? It is important to distinguish the two when interpreting their effectiveness. The **CDC** and the **CCHOS** states that respirators, such as the **N95** mask, are evaluated, tested, and approved by the **National Institute for Occupational Safety and Healthcare** and are **said** to protect against airborne particles and biological aerosols such as **bacteria and viruses**. Surgical masks, on the other hand, are cleared by the Food and Drug Administration and act simply as a barrier to splashes, droplets, spit, and other hazardous fluids. **Respirators** are said to reduce the **wearer's exposure** to particles, while **surgical masks** are **said** to protect **other people** from the wearer's respiratory emissions. Respirators are tight-fitting and are generally single use but may be used more than once, surgical masks are not tight fitting and they are for single use only (one patient encounter). **According to the CDC, surgical masks do NOT protect the wearer from inhaling airborne particles such as pathogens.**

However, other than just listening to these governing bodies, since I have already exposed their conflicts of interest, let's look at some **scientific studies** to determine if masks are even effective at all. When interpreting medical journal studies, just like interpreting whether the CDC or WHO are trustworthy, it can be consequential to consider if there are **conflicts of interest** inherent in such studies. For example, a study showing that secondhand smoke is NOT harmful, funded by a tobacco company, just might be a little bit biased, because it benefits the company's bottom line to show a favorable outcome. I did not see any major conflicts of interest declared in the studies below, but that doesn't mean they don't exist. In the example of scientific reviews published in journals on secondhand smoke, one study showed that 77% of the authors of the reviews did not disclose their sources of funding[2]. Furthermore, Richard Horton, editor of The Lancet (a peer-reviewed medical journal) stated that **perhaps half of scientific literature in general may simply be untrue** do to conflicts of interest and other problems.[3] Nevertheless, taken with a grain of salt, here we go...

Scientific Studies on Respirator/Mask-Wearing

Ann Intern Med 2020: "**Neither surgical nor cotton masks effectively filtered SARS–CoV-2 during coughs by infected patients**. Prior evidence that surgical masks effectively filtered influenza virus (1) informed recommendations that patients with confirmed or suspected COVID-19 should wear face masks to prevent transmission (2)."[4] "Oberg and Brousseau (3) demonstrated that **surgical masks did not exhibit adequate filter performance** against aerosols measuring 0.9, 2.0, and 3.1 μm in diameter. Lee and colleagues (4) showed that **particles 0.04 to 0.2 μm can penetrate surgical masks**. The size of the SARS–CoV particle from the 2002–2004 outbreak was estimated as 0.08 to 0.14 μm (5); assuming that SARS-CoV-2 has a similar size, **surgical masks are unlikely to effectively filter this virus**."[3] "This experiment did not include N95 masks".[4]

elife 2020: "Measurements of the particle filtration efficiency of N95 masks show that they are capable of filtering ≈99.8% of particles with a diameter of ≈0.1 μm [100-120 nm] (Rengasamy et al., 2017). **SARS-CoV-2 is an enveloped virus ≈0.1 μm in diameter, so N95 masks are capable of filtering most free virions**, but they do more than that. How so? Viruses are often transmitted through respiratory droplets produced by coughing and sneezing."[5] "The characteristic diameter of large droplets produced by sneezing is ~100 μm (Han et al., 2013), while the diameter of droplet nuclei produced by coughing is on the order of ~1 μm (Yang et al., 2007). At present, it is unclear whether surfaces or air are the dominant mode of SARS-CoV-2 transmission, but N95 masks should provide some protection against both (Jefferson et al., 2009; Leung et al., 2020)."[5]

ACS Nano 2020 Study: "Although the filtration efficiencies for various fabrics when a single layer was used ranged from 5 to 80% and 5 to 95% for particle sizes of <300 nm and >300 nm, respectively, the efficiencies improved when multiple layers were used and when using a specific combination of different fabrics. Filtration efficiencies of the hybrids (such as cotton-silk, cotton-chiffon, cotton-flannel) was >80% (for particles <300 nm) and >90% (for particles >300 nm). We speculate that the **enhanced performance of the hybrids** is likely due to the combined effect of mechanical and electrostatic-based filtration. **Cotton**, the most widely used material for cloth masks **performs better**

at higher weave densities (i.e., thread count) and can make a significant difference in filtration efficiencies. Our studies also imply that gaps (as caused by an **improper fit of the mask) can result in over a 60% decrease in the filtration** efficiency, implying the need for future cloth mask design studies to take into account issues of "fit" and leakage, while allowing the exhaled air to vent efficiently. Overall, we find that combinations of various commonly available fabrics used in **cloth masks can potentially provide significant protection against the transmission of aerosol particles."**[6]

BMJ 2020: "That trial, which was considered robust, **showed a benefit of masks over no masks, but no benefit of respirator masks over standard ones**, and also showed that masks were worn less than 50% of the time".[7]

"A 2010 systematic review of face masks in influenza epidemics, which included standard surgical masks and respirator masks and **found some efficacy of masks if worn by those with respiratory symptoms but not if worn by asymptomatic individuals."**[7]

"A 2007 systematic review and expert panel deliberation, which acknowledged the difficulties in interpreting evidence and stated: **"With the exception of some evidence from SARS, we did not find any published data that directly support the use of masks … by the public."**[7]

"Xiao and colleagues reviewed non-pharmaceutical measures for prevention of influenza. They identified 10 randomised controlled trials published between 1946 and 2018 that tested the efficacy of face masks (including standard surgical masks and commercially produced paper face masks designed for the public) for preventing laboratory confirmed influenza. A pooled meta-analysis **found no significant reduction in influenza transmission** (relative risk 0.78, 95% confidence interval 0.51 to 1.20; I2=30%, P=0.25). They also identified seven studies conducted in households; four provided masks for all household members, one for the sick member only, and two for household contacts only. **None showed a significant reduction in laboratory confirmed influenza in the face mask arm.** The authors concluded: **"randomized controlled trials of [face masks] did not support a substantial effect on transmission of laboratory-confirmed influenza."**[7]

"A...systematic review published on 6 April 2020 examined whether wearing a face mask or other barrier (goggles, shield, veil) prevents transmission of respiratory illness such as coronavirus, rhinovirus, tuberculosis, or influenza. It identified 31 eligible studies, including 12 randomised controlled trials. The authors found that overall, **mask wearing both in general and by infected members within households seemed to produce small but statistically non-significant reductions in infection rates.** The authors concluded that **"The evidence is not sufficiently strong to support the widespread use of facemasks as a protective measure against covid-19** and recommended further high quality randomised controlled trials."[7]

PLOS ONE 2008 Study: "Any type of general mask use is **likely to decrease viral exposure and infection risk** on a population level, in spite of imperfect fit and imperfect adherence, personal respirators providing most protection. Masks worn by patients may not offer as great a degree of protection against aerosol transmission."[8]

BMC Public Health 2007: "Other non-pharmaceutical interventions including **mask-use and other personal protective equipment for the general public, school and workplace closures early in an epidemic, and mandatory travel restrictions were rejected as likely to be ineffective, infeasible, or unacceptable to the public."**[9]

AM J Infect Control. 2009: "**Face mask use in health care workers has not been demonstrated to**

provide benefit in terms of cold symptoms or getting colds. A larger study is needed to definitively establish noninferiority of no mask use."[10]

Epidemiol. Infect. 2010: "Wearing masks incorrectly may increase the risk of transmission." "While there is some experimental evidence that masks should be able to reduce infectiousness under controlled conditions, there is less evidence on whether this translates to effectiveness in natural settings. **There is little evidence to support the effectiveness of face masks to reduce the risk of infection.**"[11]

Influenza and Other Respiratory Viruses 2011: "...one trial found a lower rate of clinical respiratory illness associated with the use of non-fit-tested N95 respirators compared with medical masks, whilst a non-inferiority trial found that masks and respirators offered similar protection to nurses against laboratory-confirmed influenza infection. A trial conducted amongst crowded, urban households found that, despite poor compliance, **mask wearing coupled with hand sanitizer use, reduced secondary transmission of upper respiratory infection/influenza-like illness/laboratory-confirmed influenza compared with education; hand sanitizer alone resulted in no reduction** in this aggregated outcome. Although **the remaining five trials found no significant differences** between control and intervention groups, there were some notable findings. **Household contacts who wore a P2 respirator** (considered to have an equivalent rating to an N95 respirator) **'all' or 'most' of the time for the first days were less likely to develop an influenza-like illness compared with less frequent users in one study.**"[12]

J Evid Based Med. 2020: "This meta-analysis showed that there were no statistically significant differences in preventing laboratory-confirmed influenza, laboratory-confirmed respiratory viral infections, laboratory-confirmed res-piratory infection and influenza-like illness using N95 respirators and surgical masks. N95 respirators provided a protective effect against laboratory-confirmed bacterial colonization."[13]

JAMA 2019: "This supports the finding that **neither N95 respirators nor medical masks were more effective in preventing laboratory-confirmed influenza or other viral respiratory infection or illness among participants when worn in a fashion consistent with current US clinical practice.**"[14]

Other Considerations

Okay. We know some differences now between types of face masks and we've seen that **the studies on respirators/masks show mixed results as to whether they work or not.** So it seems we are back to square one. Well, not exactly, because **there are many other things to think about when determining whether one should wear a mask** besides whether or not they filter viruses and/or reduce the transmission of respiratory influenza-like illnesses. For example, the Health and Safety Practices Survey of Healthcare Workers on the CDC website recommends that all workers required to wear a tight fitting respirator **have a medical evaluation to determine whether they are capable of wearing one.** Though I've maligned the CDC and the WHO, not everything they say is entirely wrong, the sentiment of some of what they say is correct and/or a good idea. I'm not saying you should go have a "medical" evaluation to determine if you are capable of wearing one, but you may want to think twice about it and, along with your practitioner, determine for yourself whether you think you are capable of wearing one. So, one question to ask yourself is, am I healthy enough to wear a mask to begin with? One should also consider that **a person aged 40-49 is probably more likely to die from car**

accidents, falling, MRSA, accidental poisoning, suicide, flu, hospital infections, stroke, cancer, and heart disease than from COVID-19.[15,16] If you are aged 40 - 49, and driving your car and going to the hospital may be more hazardous than corona, then why the big hubbub about it? Because the media chooses what it wants to focus on. On that note, I'm sure some of us have heard about the man who died in a car wreck after passing out from wearing a mask because it restricted his oxygen intake and caused a buildup of carbon dioxide in his body. Therefore, we should also inquire - **does excess CO_2 build up inside masks and is excess CO_2 bad for you? Yes, CO_2 does build up in N95 masks**, as shown by a study from 2010, published in the journal Respiratory Care.[17] And yes, **excess CO_2 is bad for you**. It is a known toxicant, can affect cognitive performance, decision making, problem resolution, cause unconsciousness, **respiratory symptoms, and respiratory arrest!**[18,19] The very things you're trying to prevent from happening from COVID! Moreover, wearing a face mask while driving, obviously increases the already higher risk of dying from driving versus COVID! **Enclosed environments are more vulnerable to CO_2 buildup** too! And what are we all being told to do? Stay inside! Stay inside your car and stay inside your homes! Meanwhile, **CO_2 levels have been rising on the planet for decades** also! At the same time all of this is going on, **5G** is being installed everywhere in America and studies have shown many harmful effects (Kostoff, 2019) and that oxygen absorbs the 60GHz frequency (Tretyakov, 2005), which may be employed in the future of 5G, so people have theorized that this **may prevent hemoglobin from effectively binding with oxygen** (plus the book *The Invisible Rainbow: A History of Electricity and Life* correlates that the occurrence of epidemics/pandemics often come soon after large scale new electrical devices/networks have been set up on Earth). To put a cherry on top of the mounds of evidence here and the heaps of mask cream piling up at landfills and polluting the planet everywhere, **one of the major complications that leads to a person's death from COVID-19 is hypoxia** (a lack of oxygen because the lungs fill up with fluid) (Huang, 2020). It sure sounds like there's a giant conspiracy to induce hypoxic hysteria on the masses to me. I might die of irony overload writing this, or perhaps all the iron I'm accumulating will save me by building more red blood cells to carry more oxygen in my body. Or I could just not wear a mask, wear some EMF blocking clothing, take some natural dietary supplements, and eat healthily and maybe I'll be spared of the perilous plague possibly perpetrated upon us! Whew! I'm a little out of breath now after all that. Anyway, jokes aside, if the man who died in the car wreck's family members are aware of these facts, the irony of them in relation to the tragic fate of the man, they are likely to be haunted and guilt-ridden by them forever. Not to mention, **the number of cases of COVID-19 and the death rates from COVID-19 are inflated** anyway due to the fact that some of the tests do not actually test for the SARS-CoV-2 virus, the virus that causes COVID-19, and due to the fact that they are classifying deaths as COVID-19 deaths if a person came into contact with somebody who had COVID-19, but did not necessarily die from COVID-19. As Deborah Birx, one of the physicians leading the White House's Coronavirus Task Force said, "We've taken a very liberal approach to mortality". **Coronaviruses are among the most frequent causes of the common cold** (Paules et al.). What else should we take into account about masks? Well, it turns out there are other detrimental health effects of wearing them. One study showed an **increase in headaches** of participants wearing masks.[10] Another showed a potential for development of **skin lesions, irritant dermatitis, or worsening acne** when used frequently for long hours.[20] There's a **potential increased risk of self-contamination due to the manipulation of a face mask**.[21, 22] Difficulty breathing and tiredness may be caused by mask-wearing (Kim et al.), (Esposito et al.). And **what about inhaling bleach**? The CDC recommends either washing face masks in your washing machine with your other laundry or hand washing them with bleach. The WHO recommends pretty much the same thing but says when you can't use hot water, then either boil the mask or use .1% chlorine then thoroughly rinse the mask afterward. If one doesn't have hot water or a washing machine, then one ought to ask themselves, **which is riskier, the possibility of catching**

coronavirus, or inhaling chlorine bleach every day for the past 6 months that this virus has been around and well into the future? "Chlorine gas is a potent pulmonary irritant that causes acute damage in both the upper and lower respiratory tract."[23] Still, there's more. **Should the same face mask recommendations be given across the board depending on the state one lives in? Does one's blood type reduce their risk of infection? What affect does temperature and humidity have on the coronavirus? What other precautionary measures is a person taking besides wearing a mask? Are masks and hand sanitizers the only way to protect oneself from infection and complications from infection? Are they the best ways? Is one weakening one's immune system by filtering out healthy bacteria and viruses in the air? Does relying solely on a mask and hand sanitizer give a person a false sense of security that leads them to not take other more important precautionary measures against the virus?** Let's answer these questions too. **In Florida, we live in a very hot and humid state**. Preliminary evidence published in 2020 showed that **higher temperatures are associated with lower incidence of COVID-19**.[24] In March, Live Science posted an article that stated that 90% of Coronavirus infections occurred in areas between 37.4 and 62.6 degrees Fahrenheit. Less than 6% of global cases occurred in countries with an average temperature above 64.4 degrees and an absolute humidity above 9 g/m3. Some researchers have gone so far as to propose a weather pattern that COVID-19 follows along called the Corona Belt. Influenza is always more prominent in the winter-time due to drier and colder weather. Shaman et al. demonstrated in a study[25] from 2010 that absolute **humidity is likely the predominant determinant of influenza seasonality**. There are other sides to this coin, though. Florida was ranked 18th in the country for per capita (per 100 people) COVID cases as of April, 2020 and 19th in case fatality rate in May, 2020. Not great, but not terrible either. But, we do have a lot of old people. The state rankings you see on T.V. are not usually per capita, just the amount of cases for the whole state. Some states are bigger than others. Does blood type increase or decrease one's risk of COVID-19? A non-peer-reviewed pre-print of a study from 2020 showed that blood group A is associated with an increased risk of COVID-19 and blood group O is associated with a decreased risk (Zhao, 2020). Roughly 40% of Americans have type O blood. What other measures is a person or business taking besides wearing or mandating masks to employees and are they better than masks? **Some health food stores run an ozonator daily** to purify the air. Ozone is an eco-friendly, yet powerful trioxygen disinfectant that is produced naturally within Earth's atmosphere. It can oxidize anything including viruses, bacteria, and organic and inorganic molecules. Some health food stores know to tightly control the levels of ozone in the store to purify the air in a safe and healthy fashion. Some retail vitamin shops are in the process of installing **UV light** within their air conditioning system to purify the air. Nearly all stores currently offer **curbside service** for those who do not wish to go inside. Some health food stores use tiny amounts of hydrogen peroxide in their cleaning solution and **sanitize carts and baskets at the front door. 6 foot social distancing measures are in place** with floor markings at most businesses. At this time, many stores are making it **mandatory for at least a portion of their employees to wear masks** as well. And, last but not least, if you shop at a local health food store for your groceries and natural medicine, then you may be taking less of a risk than shopping at some big box store. This is because the other customers who shop at a health food store are likely eating healthily and taking natural immune boosting supplements, possibly reducing the chances of infection and the spreading germs. For example, olive leaf extract has been shown to reduce viral shedding (Renis et al., Micol et al.). I think we've answered a few questions with those last sentences but I can't answer them all. But let's ask some more shall we!? Questioning the allopathic, conventional, big pharma, medical model recommendations and the mainstream media's narrative is, after all, probably one of the healthiest things we can do when it comes to this "pandemic". Some of the questions below are borrowed from an article by Denis G. Rancourt, PhD.

Unknown Aspects and Unanswered Questions of Mask-Wearing:

Does a community of natural health-minded people have the same risk for the spread of infection as the general public?

Should the government be in charge of your health or you?

Do used masks become sources of enhanced transmission, for the wearer and others?

Do masks collect and retain pathogens that the mask wearer would otherwise avoid when breathing naturally without a mask?

Are large droplets caught by a mask atomized or aerosolized into inhalable components?

Can virions escape an evaporating droplet stuck to a face mask?

What are the dangers of bacterial growth on a used mask?

How do pathogen-laden droplets interact with other environmental particles captured on the mask?

What are the long-term health effects of impeded breathing?

Are there negative social consequences to a masked society?

Are there negative psychological consequences to wearing a mask, as a fear-based behavioral modification?

What are the environmental consequences of mask manufacturing and disposal?

Do the masks shed fibres or substances that are harmful when inhaled?'

Summary: What Have We Learned?

- Wearing or not wearing a mask is a personal choice and nobody should be shamed for making either choice

- Government agencies claim that N95 respirators are different than surgical masks and claim that they offer more protection for the wearer against viruses

- Surgical masks are for single, one patient/person encounter use only and are only claimed to offer minor protection for other people of one's respiratory emissions and are not claimed to protect a wearer against viruses

- Some studies show that respirators/masks work and some studies show they don't work

- Respirators might work better than surgical masks or not or neither of them work

- An improperly fitted mask may increase the risk of transmission or it may not

- Half of the scientific literature may be fraudulent

- The science is NEVER settled

- Bill Gates has given the CDC and WHO a lot of money which may cause conflicts of interest in their recommendations

- Getting vaccinated with a flu vaccine may possibly increase one's risk of being infected with coronaviruses and vaccines may not be healthy for you

- A simulated coronavirus outbreak called Event 201 was staged and funded by The Bill and Melinda Gates Foundation roughly one month prior to the actual outbreak

- Pandemics/epidemics may possibly coincide with new large scale electromagnetic devices/networks being set up on Earth

- One may need to have a medical evaluation to determine if one is healthy enough to wear a mask

- A person aged 40-49 is more likely to die from car accidents, falling, MRSA, accidental poisoning, suicide, flu, hospital infections, stroke, cancer, and heart disease than from COVID-19

- COVID-19 death rates are inflated

- Coronaviruses are among the most frequent causes of the common cold

- Florida is a hot, humid state and higher temps and higher humidity is associated with less incidence of COVID-19

- Blood type may play a role in one's risk of contracting COVID-19

- There are other precautions one can take to bolster one's health besides mask-wearing

- Some health food stores purify their air with ozone

- Some vitamin shops are installing UV light in their A/C system to kill pathogens

- Some health food stores disinfect carts and baskets

- Many businesses apply social distancing measures with floor markings

- Many stores already make it mandatory for at least a portion of their employees to wear masks

- Health food stores sell antiviral dietary supplements and healthy food

- **There are detrimental health consequences of wearing masks such as:**

- Difficulty breathing

- Increased headaches

- Elevated CO_2 levels

- Maybe more likely to die in a car while wearing a mask

- Inhaling of toxic bleach

- Skin lesions, irritant dermatitis, or worsening acne has been documented in studies on wearing masks

- Potential increased risk of self-contamination from wearing a mask

- Tiredness

- The jury is still out as to whether masks work or not and blindly accepting that they work may put one more at risk due to having a false sense of security, while not taking other important precautions

- There are unanswered questions if masks have other detrimental effects

- It is probably healthy to question the allopathic, conventional, medical model recommendations and the mainstream media's narrative and stance on masks, but you should always talk to your doctor/naturopath/practitioner before making any changes/decisions

Hopefully all of this information I have presented you with puts your mind and lungs at ease when going out in public. I appreciate your patronage and believe that I am going above and beyond and taking more than adequate precautionary measures to ensure the safety and health of myself and others. You are responsible for your own health and your own decisions. I am not liable whether you choose to wear a mask or not. I only present information for your consideration. You should always talk to your doctor or holistic practitioner before making any changes. If you have other questions about what you can do to support your immune system in this challenging time, I have other protocols I have created that are either free or available for purchase on my website and I am equipped with the skill and knowledge to assist you in a consultation if you would like one. Breathe easy.

These statements have not been evaluated by the FDA. This article is not an attempt to treat, diagnose, prevent, or cure any disease or condition. Talk to your doctor before making any changes.

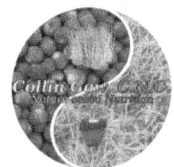

References:
1. Wolff GG. Influenza vaccination and respiratory virus interference among Department of Defense personnel during the 2017-2018 influenza season. Vaccine. 2020;38(2):350-354. doi:10.1016/j.vaccine.2019.10.005
2. Barnes DE, Bero LA. Why review articles on the health effects of passive smoking reach different conclusions. JAMA. 1998;279(19):1566-1570. doi:10.1001/jama.279.19.1566
3. Gyles C. Skeptical of medical science reports?. Can Vet J. 2015;56(10):1011-1012.
4. Bae S, Kim MC, Kim JY, et al. Effectiveness of Surgical and Cotton Masks in Blocking SARS-CoV-2: A Controlled Comparison in 4 Patients [published online ahead of print, 2020 Apr 6] [retracted in: Ann Intern Med. 2020 Jun 2;:]. Ann Intern Med. 2020;M20-1342. doi:10.7326/M20-1342
5. Bar-On YM, Flamholz A, Phillips R, Milo R. SARS-CoV-2 (COVID-19) by the numbers. Elife. 2020;9:e57309. Published 2020 Apr 2. doi:10.7554/eLife.57309

6. Konda A, Prakash A, Moss GA, Schmoldt M, Grant GD, Guha S. Aerosol Filtration Efficiency of Common Fabrics Used in Respiratory Cloth Masks. ACS Nano. 2020;14(5):6339-6347. doi:10.1021/acsnano.0c03252

7. Greenhalgh Trisha, Schmid Manuel B, Czypionka Thomas, Bassler Dirk, Gruer Laurence. Face masks for the public during the covid-19 crisis BMJ 2020; 369 :m1435

8. van der Sande M, Teunis P, Sabel R. Professional and home-made face masks reduce exposure to respiratory infections among the general population. PLoS One. 2008;3(7):e2618. Published 2008 Jul 9. doi:10.1371/journal.pone.0002618

9. Aledort JE, Lurie N, Wasserman J, Bozzette SA. Non-pharmaceutical public health interventions for pandemic influenza: an evaluation of the evidence base. BMC Public Health. 2007;7:208. Published 2007 Aug 15. doi:10.1186/1471-2458-7-208

10. Jacobs JL, Ohde S, Takahashi O, Tokuda Y, Omata F, Fukui T. Use of surgical face masks to reduce the incidence of the common cold among health care workers in Japan: a randomized controlled trial. Am J Infect Control. 2009;37(5):417-419. doi:10.1016/j.ajic.2008.11.002

11. COWLING, B. J., ZHOU, Y., IP, D. K. M., LEUNG, G. M., & AIELLO, A. E. (2010). Face masks to prevent transmission of influenza virus: a systematic review. Epidemiology and Infection, 138(04), 449. doi:10.1017/s0950268809991658

12. Bin-Reza, Faisal & Lopez Chavarrias, Vicente & Nicoll, Angus & Chamberland, Mary. (2011). The use of masks and respirators to prevent transmission of influenza: A systematic review of the scientific evidence. Influenza and other respiratory viruses. 6. 257-67. 10.1111/j.1750-2659.2011.00307.x.

13. Long Y, Hu T, Liu L, et al. Effectiveness of N95 respirators versus surgical masks against influenza: A systematic review and meta-analysis. J Evid Based Med. 2020;13(2):93-101. doi:10.1111/jebm.12381

14. Radonovich LJ Jr, Simberkoff MS, Bessesen MT, et al. N95 Respirators vs Medical Masks for Preventing Influenza Among Health Care Personnel: A Randomized Clinical Trial. JAMA. 2019;322(9):824-833. doi:10.1001/jama.2019.11645

15. All accidental death information from National Safety Council. Disease death information from Centers for Disease Control and Prevention. Shark fatality data provided by the International Shark Attack File. Lifetime risk is calculated by dividing 2003 population (290,850,005) by the number of deaths, divided by 77.6, the life expectancy of a person born in 2003.

16. The Epidemiological Characteristics of an Outbreak of 2019 Novel Coronavirus Diseases (COVID-19) - China CCDC, February 17 2020. Report of the WHO-China Joint Mission on Coronavirus Disease 2019 (COVID-19) [Pdf] - World Health Organization, Feb. 28, 2020.

17. Roberge RJ, Coca A, Williams WJ, Powell JB, Palmiero AJ. Physiological impact of the N95 filtering facepiece respirator on healthcare workers. Respir Care. 2010;55(5):569-577.

18. Azuma, K., Kagi, N., Yanagi, U., & Osawa, H. (2018). Effects of low-level inhalation exposure to carbon dioxide in indoor environments: A short review on human health and psychomotor performance. Environment International, 121, 51–56. doi:10.1016/j.envint.2018.08.059

19. Permentier K, Vercammen S, Soetaert S, Schellemans C. Carbon dioxide poisoning: a literature review of an often forgotten cause of intoxication in the emergency department. Int J Emerg Med. 2017;10(1):14. doi:10.1186/s12245-017-0142-y

20. Al Badri F. Surgical mask contact dermatitis and epidemiology of contact dermatitis in healthcare workers. . Current Allergy & Clinical Immunology, 30,3: 183 - 188. 2017.

21. Zamora JE, Murdoch J, Simchison B, Day AG. Contamination: a comparison of 2 personal protective systems. CMAJ. 2006;175(3):249-54.

22. Kwon JH, Burnham CD, Reske KA, Liang SY, Hink T, Wallace MA, et al. Assessment of Healthcare Worker Protocol Deviations and Self-Contamination During Personal Protective Equipment

Donning and Doffing. Infect Control Hosp Epidemiol. 2017;38(9):1077-83.

23. Akdur O, Durukan P, Ikizceli I, Ozkan S, Avsarogullari L. A rare complication of chlorine gas inhalation: pneumomediastinum. Emerg Med J. 2006;23(11):e59. doi:10.1136/emj.2006.040022

24. Bannister-Tyrrell, Melanie & Meyer, Anne & Faverjon, Céline & Cameron, Angus. (2020). Preliminary evidence that higher temperatures are associated with lower incidence of COVID-19, for cases reported globally up to 29th February 2020. 10.1101/2020.03.18.20036731.

25. Shaman J, Pitzer VE, Viboud C, Grenfell BT, Lipsitch M. Absolute humidity and the seasonal onset of influenza in the continental United States [published correction appears in PLoS Biol. 2010;8(3). doi: 10.1371/annotation/35686514-b7a9-4f65-9663-7baefc0d63c0]. PLoS Biol. 2010;8(2):e1000316. Published 2010 Feb 23. doi:10.1371/journal.pbio.1000316

Protocols

Black mold (*Stachybotrys chartarum*) is a common type of cellulolytic, saprophytic, filamentous yeast/fungi found in indoor air samples. However, many types of molds have been found as well, the most common being *Cladosporium*, *Penicillium*, *Aspergillus*, and *Alternaria*, according to the C.D.C.. Over 80 genera of fungi have been associated with respiratory allergies, however. Many of these molds can contribute to "Sick Building Syndrome". **People in developed countries spend over 90% of their time indoors** (Cincinelli et al.). The most important step to treating mold problems is to get outside! One study stated, "avoidance of exposure is the most effective mode of therapy" (Bitnun et al.). Fungal contamination of indoor environments **may cause headaches, allergies, asthma, irritant effects, eye ailments, respiratory problems, mycoses (fungal diseases), skin rashes, dizziness, nausea, immunosuppression, autoimmunity, neuropathy, chronic fatigue, idiopathic pulmonary hemorrhage in infants, diarrhea, sore throat, and several other symptoms and health problems**. Allergies are the most common reaction to molds. When trying to eradicate mold from your body, besides taking anti-fungals to kill the mold, it's important to support your liver, lymphatic system, and bowels to cleanse the mold toxins out of your system and to prevent too many side effects from all the strong anti-fungals. I have highlighted some of my favorites for mold issues below. Pick 3 or 4 options.

Tests: Vasoactive Intestinal Polypeptide, Melanocyte Stimulating Hormone, TGF Beta-1 - Transforming Growth Factor Beta-1, **C4a**, HLA DR, AGA IgA/IgG, ACTH/Cortisol, VEGF, ACLA IgA/IgG/IgM, ADH/Osmolality, MMP-9, Leptin, Nasal Culture, and ERMI testing are all possible tests you may need to confirm mold illness. Survivingmold.com is a good resource to learn more about these tests.

Biofilm busters: Many types of fungi and bacteria create biofilms to protect themselves from your immune system. Attacking biofilms may help antifungal agents to work better. **NAC**, EDTA, **serrapeptase**, pomegranate, berberine, green tea, cloves, quercetin, ginger, ginkgo, cranberry, green tea, rosemary, magnolia bark, L. paracasei, L. rhamnosus, and L. fermentum, have all shown anti-biofilm activity. **Anti-fungals: oregano oil**, **garlic**, boswellia, black walnut, wormwood, caprylic acid, burdock, acerola, pau d'arco, **grapefruit seed extract**, **silver**, berberine, goldenseal, olive leaf, ashwagandha, turmeric, manuka honey, **propolis**, aloe, pomegranate, cinnamon, and chilis. Among 5 commercially available disinfectants, **tea trea oil** had the strongest inhibitory effect against *Aspergillus fumigatus* and *Penicillium chrysogenum* in oil or vapor form (Rogawansamy et al.). **Clove oil** was strongest among essential oils in another study against fungi collected from indoor air samples (Schroder et al.). **Black seed oil** has been studied for a number of respiratory ailments and has strong anti-fungal activity (Yimer et al.). **Cholestyramine** and **Charcoal bind biotoxins** in the small intestine (do not take cholestyramine if you have low cholesterol, as this medication can also bind cholesterol).

Immune strengthening: zinc, vitamin A, vitamin E, vitamin C, selenium, vitamin D3, **probiotics**, prebiotics, echinacea, andrographis, elderberry, aloe, olive leaf, lysine, plant sterols, etc. **Liver cleansers: glutathione**, sulforaphane, **NAC**, calcium d-glucarate, DIM, turmeric, dandelion, artichoke, **milk thistle**, alpha lipoic acid, **fiber**, methionine, beet root, schizandra, licorice. **Lymphatic cleansers: echinacea**, burdock, red clover, yellow dock, dandelion, MSM. **Allergies: quercetin**, zinc, vitamin D3, nettles, L-histidine, saline/gse/oregano/silver nasal spray. **Respiratory: Nebulize glutathione or silver**.

Home/Lifestyle: Buy a de-humidifier for your house, as molds like moisture. **Diffuse essential oils. Get a HEPA air filter and/or ozonator.** Try an **infra red sauna. Buy salt lamps. Try dry brushing. Avoid refined foods, carbs, and sugars. Temporarily reduce carbohydrates and sugars in the diet** when addressing mold toxicity, as fungi feed on sugar.

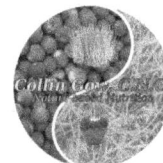

Bloating (Digestive)

Digestive tract bloating may be caused by **indigestion** from **low stomach acid** or **insufficient pancreatic enzyme production, liver and gallbladder congestion, SIBO** (small intestinal bacterial overgrowth) due to past antibiotic or acid reflux medication use, **Candida overgrowth, G.I. dysbiosis, unhealthy, refined, or high protein/high fat foods**, or other problems. Bloating may cause pain, discomfort, and distension of the abdomen as well as inflammation of the G.I. Tract from improperly digested foods. Water weight bloating is different from digestive bloating.

Increase stomach acid with 1 Tablespoon **apple cider vinegar** with mother in 3 ounces of water two times per day in the middle of two largest meals or try 2 teaspoons of **Swedish bitters** with main meals. **Potassium, iodine, chloride, b-vitamins, and any bitter or spicy herbs** may assist with stomach acid production and/or secretion. Stomach acid in pill form may be taken as **HCL** instead of apple cider vinegar, if desired, though I do not usually recommend it, as it is not as safe, nor as healthy.

Take a **digestive enzyme** at the beginning of each main meal or try **Dr. Chi G.I. Chi** and **Digestron**.

Try carminative herbs (herbs known to help expel gas from the intestinal tract): Try 4 oz **peppermint, ginger, or fennel tea** double brewed with meals. **Add cumin, anise, or caraway** to foods. **Peppermint softgels** or **charcoal** are other good options. **Antispasmodic herbs** may help as well, such as **lobelia, chamomile, skullcap, valerian, kava, cramp bark, wild oats, Jamaican dogwood,** etc.

Take a multi-mineral and/or trace mineral product. Minerals are the precursors to enzymes, as they are necessary to produce enzymes. Enzymes are metalloproteins, meaning every enzyme requires a metallic ion cofactor to be produced and function in the body.

Take a probiotic supplement and eat fermented foods. Probiotics containing soil-based organisms may be especially helpful for bloating, however, they are strong, they are not for everyone, and they should not necessarily be taken every day or long term.

Get tested for SIBO. Peppermint softgels or **Atrantil** may be useful for SIBO.

Get tested for Candida or perform a Candida self-test. The method is as follows: spit into a full cup of water and let sit overnight. If tendrils or root like structures form, then you may have candida overgrowth. A thick white coating on the tongue may also confirm Candidiasis. Antifungals such as **oregano oil, black walnut, garlic, olive leaf, boswellia, propolis, caprylic acid, tea tree oil, grapefruit seed extract, pau d'arco,** and others may be useful for killing Candida.

Reduce grains, legumes (beans, chickpeas, peas, lentils, peanuts, cashews), and corn. Eat gluten free. Reduce portion sizes of meat, cheese, or any such rich foods high in protein and/or fat. **Do not consume oils or other refined foods. Do not consume more than 6 ounces of liquid with meals. Eat papaya and pineapple** for papain and bromelain. **Eat artichokes** for the liver/gallbladder. **Eat dandelion greens** for bitters. **Eat fermented foods** such as kimchi, sauerkraut, umeboshi plums, tempeh, miso, kombucha, or goat milk kefir. Press on the ileocecal valve and/or valve of Houston (located 1 inch below and 2 – 3 inches to the left and right of the belly button) or, turned sideways, try bending over at the waist a few times.

These statements have not been evaluated by the FDA. This is not an attempt to treat, diagnose, prevent, or cure any disease or condition. Talk to your doctor before making any changes.

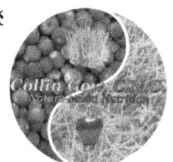

Blood Pressure

Hypertension (high blood pressure) is the greatest risk factor for heart disease and stroke. **Heart disease is the #1 killer in America**. In 2017 the AHA came out with new blood pressure guidelines, the first since 2003. Stage 1 hypertension is now considered as a blood pressure between 130-139/80-89. **High BP may be caused by caffeine consumption, choline deficiency, anxiety, stress, alcohol consumption, kidney disease/nephritis, insulin resistance, cadmium toxicity, excess sodium and insufficient potassium, or other causes**. The HPA axis, the autonomic nervous system, the kidneys, thyroid, and other systems in the body help to regulate blood pressure. Pick 2 or 3 options below.

Beet juice contains naturally occurring nitrates, which may increase nitric oxide. Nitric oxide is a vasodilator (opens up the blood vessels), which may assist healthy blood pressure levels. Try 3 Tablespoons twice per day, Spinach is also high in nitrates.

1 Tbsp **Apple cider vinegar** in 3oz water twice per day with meals may help with healthy blood pressure levels.

Garlic thins the blood by lowering fibrinogen levels and may act as a natural ACE inhibitor. High fibrinogen and high ACE have been associated with an increased risk of hypertension. Eat ½ a clove of raw garlic twice per day or try 4 garlic capsules per day (Do not take if already on a blood thinner). **Pomegranate** and **Lactobacillus helveticus** from fermented dairy are other natural ACE inhibitors.

Olive leaf, arginine, citrulline, celery seed, taurine, magnesium, hawthorn, bitter melon, nattokinase (be careful with if on a blood thinner), msm, grapeseed extract, COQ10, iodine, GABA, borage oil, cacao, serine, choline, berberine, reishi, vitamin C, carnosine, histidine, propolis, vitamin D, Lactobacillus plantarum, and germanium are other good choices for healthy blood pressure levels. **Taurine and magnesium may reduce stress**. Stress can cause high blood pressure. **Taurine** opposes adrenaline, acting like a natural beta blocker and **mag** acts as a natural calcium channel blocker and vasodilator and relaxes the nerves and muscles, melting away tension.

Eat a whole food, plant-based diet consisting of lots of fruits and vegetables. **Eat watermelon**, it's high in citrulline, which may convert into nitric oxide. **Oats** or **oat bran** are good for those who can tolerate grains. Their high **fiber** content may be beneficial for high blood pressure. Other high fiber foods include fruits, veggies, beans, lentils, seeds, and roots/tubers. Cook roots/tubers and veggies al dente, rather than cooking them to mush. Eat **celery**. **Drink fresh coconut water.** It's high potassium content may be important to balance blood pressure. Other **potassium** rich foods are helpful, especially potatoes, sweet potatoes, purple potatoes, beet tops, and citrus fruits (**do not increase potassium if on a potassium sparing diuretic such as amiloride, eplerenone, spironolactone, triamterene or if on a prescription ACE inhibitor, NSAID, or ARB medication**). Use dulse, celery salt, or **garlic granules** in place of salt. Consume **5oz goat kefir** twice per week. Fermented dairy may reduce the risk of hypertension. **Parsley, dandelion leaves, and cranberries** are good to eat as well. They are natural diuretics. **Breathe, de-stress, and exercise.**

Available for download @ collingowcnc.wixsite.com/collingowcnc/articlesandprotocols

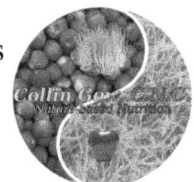

Cholesterol

Cholesterol is a naturally occurring, waxy, steroid precursor **produced by the body in response to inflammation** in the blood vessels but is **also a necessary raw material and backbone from which hormones like vitamin D, pregnenolone, DHEA, cortisol, testosterone, estrogen, and progesterone are made**. It's also important for cell membrane health, myelin, (the protective coating of nerves) and the brain. More important than the total number of cholesterol is the ratio of oxidized LDL cholesterol (bad cholesterol) to HDL cholesterol (good cholesterol). High HDL is correlated with a low risk of heart disease. There are also different types of LDL. LDL-A are large lipoprotein molecules that are less likely to stick to arteries than LDL-B. **Ask your doctor for an LDL subfractions test or LDL particle test to determine your LDL-A and LDL-B levels**. The body has a daily requirement for 1g of cholesterol for the production of hormones. This can be manufactured by the body if healthy. **Cholesterol that's too low (below 160mg/dL) is not good either. It may increase risk of stroke, depression, suicide, violent behavior, lung ailments, cancer, and alcoholism**. The liver plays the primary role in removing cholesterol from the body by metabolizing it and dumping it into the gallbladder. The gallbladder then releases it into the intestines and it comes out in stool. **Tobacco smoking, alcohol, hyperinsulinemia, excessive carbohydrates, fructose, trans fatty acids, stress, butter, and coconut oil may raise total cholesterol**.

Choline, B6, and inositol are necessary for the **metabolism of cholesterol**.

Turmeric is great for reducing **inflammation**. Inflammation may increase cholesterol levels.

Artichoke is a cholagogue and cholerectic (**helps with the production and flow of bile**). It's great for activating the gallbladder which may help to release cholesterol and its Cynarin content may help with healthy cholesterol levels.

Amla is a high antioxidant superfruit berry also called Indian gooseberry. Recent research indicates it may be beneficial for maintaining healthy blood sugar and cholesterol levels. **Guggul** is a gum resin from the guggul tree that assists with high cholesterol by **converting LDL into HDL** through the liver, improving thyroid health, and **inhibiting the production of cholesterol**.

Bergamot**,** green tea, cinnamon, berberine, resveratrol, red yeast rice, OPCs, spirulina, cumin, alpha-linolenic acid, linoleic acid, charcoal, vitamin C, arginine, cacao, garlic, and acacia gum **may all have beneficial effects on cholesterol levels**.

Plant sterols such as Beta sitosterol, campesterol, sitostanol, and stigmasterol, as well as psyllium, galactomannans, sesame lignans, sesame seeds, alginates, gamma oryzanol, rice bran, legumes, fish oils, eggplant, alfalfa, chilis, and lecithin **all reduce the absorption of dietary cholesterol**.

Eat artichokes, apples, pomegranates, oranges, blackberries, broccoli sprouts, onions, and celery. Consume **flax, chia, walnuts, savi seeds, hemp seeds, and hemp milk. Eat oatmeal** if you can tolerate grains. **Eat a more whole food, plant-based diet** consisting of lots of fruits and vegetables (reduce animal foods to 1 serving or less per day). **Increase fiber in your diet**. Sweet potatoes and purple potatoes cooked al dente (and eat the skin too), fruits, vegetables, beans, lentils, nuts, seeds, and whole grains are good options. **Use oils only sparingly**, but when using, choose olive oil, walnut oil, or hemp oil. Out of these 3, only cook with olive oil or no oil and cook at low temp.

These statements have not been evaluated by the FDA. This is not an attempt to treat, diagnose, prevent, or cure any disease or condition. Talk to your doctor before making any changes.

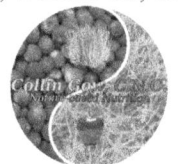

Energy

True energy comes from getting extremely healthy. The simple way to do that is to get a lot of nutrition, which detoxifies the bad and builds up the good. Consuming **lots of fruits and veggies, super foods,** getting at least **8 hours of sleep** and getting enough **electrolytes** are all important for energy and overall health. 70% of the brain's energy is derived from carbohydrates, while 70% of the heart's energy is derived from fats. The brain can use medium chain triglycerides, glutamine, and postbiotics/SCFAs as fuel sources, however, as well. Pick 2 or 3 options below for a pick me up!

Supplements

Thyroid: Iodine, tyrosine, and selenium after breakfast. These are important for a properly functioning thyroid. The thyroid is a key regulator of metabolism (energy). Tyrosine is also important to raise adrenaline if there's an adrenaline deficiency. Adrenaline breaks down body fat and turns it into energy. **Vitamin C** is necessary for the synthesis of tyrosine from phenylalanine.

Adrenals: Licorice, rhodiola, schizandra, astragalus, maca, eleuthero, ginseng, and cordyceps boost adrenal function, which may help to balance energy and stress. Licorice is unique amongst these as it raises cortisol, blood sugar, and blood pressure. Some people need this for energy.

Mitochondrial Boosters: COQ10, PQQ, Ribose, Carnitine, Alpha Lipoic Acid, and **Nicotinamide or NAD.** The mitochondria is the energy center of your cells where energy is produced in the form of **Adenosine Triphosphate (ATP).** These supplements may enhance the mitochondria's metabolism of fats, proteins, or carbs, or increase the number of mitochondria, facilitating energy production.

Minerals: Iron (especially for women). Iron deficiency is the #1 most common nutrient deficiency in the world. Women usually respond well to iron for energy. It helps build the blood, oxygenate the body, and raise metabolism. **Copper** is essential to produce Cytochrome C Oxidase. The reduction in this enzyme is said to be responsible for age related decreases in energy. Oxidation is integral for the production of energy. Iron, copper, and iodine are **pro-oxidants.**

Aminos: Glutamine and Aspartic acid. Glutamine acts as an excitatory amino acid in the nervous system if taken on an empty stomach. This will help wake up your brain and body. With food it will convert into GABA and calm you. So be sure to do it on an empty stomach. Aspartic acid raises energy.

Vitamins: B-complex. All B-vitamins help convert food into energy, not just b12.

Oils: Peppermint oil may help with nervous exhaustion and better blood flow to the brain.

Foods/Lifestyle

Superfoods like **Spirulina, Chlorella, or Blue green algae** are good. Spirulina is higher in protein than beef. It is also the highest source of tyrosine in nature besides kelp. Tyrosine may increase motivation. **Sour foods** are important sources of organic acids. Your entire Krebs cycle (energy production cycle/citric acid cycle) is a combination of organic acids. **Eat citrus fruits, green apples, raspberries,** etc. **Green tea, matcha, yerba mate, or black coffee** for caffeine. **Dark chocolate** for theobromine (a caffeine related compound). Consume enough **protein** (.8g/kg of body weight). Potassium may increase endurance. **Bananas, coconut water, sweet potatoes, purple potatoes, fruit, and beet tops** are high in it. **Get enough calcium**, it's a key electrolyte also. **Calcium fortified plant milks** are good. Eat **balanced meals** that contain fats, proteins, carbs, and fiber. **Get hormones checked.** Low Testosterone may reduce energy.

Available for download @ collingowcnc.wixsite.com/collingowcnc/articlesandprotocols

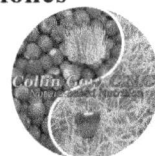

Healthy Cell Growth—8 Phases

Abnormal cell growth contributes to the second leading cause of death in America. It may occur as a result of **infection** from different pathogens such as viruses (Masrour-Roudsari, Ebrahimpour et al.), bacteria (Masrour-Roudsari, Ebrahimpour et al.), fungi (Faden et al.), or protozoa (De Flora, La Maestra et al.), **mitochondrial/metabolic conditions** (Seyfried et al.), **genetic defects** (Campbell et al.), **diet and lifestyle** (Gupta, Kim, Aggarwal et al.), **inflammation** (Coussens, Werb et al.), **oxidative stress** (Liu, Ren, Zhang...et al.), a **weakened immune system** (Corthay et al.), **hypoxia** (oxygen deficiency) (Moen, Stuhr et al.), **improper cooking** (John, Stern, Koo et al.), (Joshi, Kim, Stern et al.), (Anderson, Sinha, Kulldorff,...et al.), **obesity** (Pergola, Silvestris et al.), **environmental contaminants/pollutants** (Koriech et al.), **radiation exposure** (Shah, Sachs, Wilson et al.), **high insulin** (Thomas, Rome, Ujvari et al.), (Pustylnikov, Costabile, Beghi...et al.), **high or low cholesterol** (Kitahara, González, Freedman...et al.), and/or **hormonal imbalances** (Parkin et al.), (Sherbet et al.), (Travis, Key et al.), and so on. There are many things to consider in one's effort to maintain healthy cell growth. The **5 categories** I tend to emphasize are: 1. Remain alkaline, 2. Supercharge the immune system, 3. Detoxify, 4. Reduce exposure to and detoxify xenoestrogens specifically, and 5. Eat a more whole food, organic, raw, plant-based diet. It's also necessary to know and support each phase of the formation and spread of abnormal cells. These **8 phases** include 1. Inflammation/oxidative stress leading to damaged mitochondria and mutation of DNA, 2. Anaerobic and/or Aerobic Glycolysis due to hypoxia and ROS damaged mitochondria 3. Abnormal stem cell production, 4. Angiogenesis, 5. Survival, 6. Growth, 7. Metastasis and invasion. **These particular sheets only designate and discuss healthy options to address these <u>phases</u> that abnormal cells undergo.** I have also included some other random information about healthy cell growth on the last page of these sheets, such as how to increase the effectiveness of cytotoxic allopathic treatments for abnormal cells, reduce their toxicity, and mitigate their side effects, should one decide to go that route for treatment. **Be sure to pick up the other sheets on healthy cell growth for more information.**

1. Inflammation/Oxidative stress: There are a myriad of causes of inflammation/oxidative stress, many of them are listed above already within the second sentence on this page. A few others are inadequate sleep, excessive exercise, high mental or physical stress, and many many others. The fact is, simply living, breathing, and eating, and basically just about anything and everything for that matter can cause inflammation and oxidative stress. Of course, choosing healthy ways to eat and live and breathe do help, however. Elevated **reactive oxygen species (ROS aka free radicals aka oxidants)** is an important way to describe inflammation/oxidative stress. Elevated ROS are implicated in a number of diseases, inflammatory conditions, and abnormal cell development, including initiation, promotion, progression, and growth, (Liu, Ren, Zhang...et al.). Interestingly, moderately elevated **ROS** leads to **mutations** and abnormal cell development, yet inducing ROS in high levels may lead to apoptosis (cell suicide) in abnormal cells once they have already formed. Apoptosis of unhealthy cells is a good thing. However, inducing high ROS may also kill healthy cells or cause healthy cells to transform into abnormal ones. This double edge sword and dual role of ROS is important to balance. Redox homeostasis is the best way to balance ROS - this is what antioxidant supplements actually do. Almost all antioxidants do not function as "antioxidants". Instead, they perform redox homeostasis via mimicking oxidants (also called electrophiles in redox lingo), yet they do not cause harm, (Ursini, Maiorino, Forman et al.), (Forman, Davies, Ursini et al.). This oxidant mimicking by antioxidants stimulates an increase in endogenous antioxidant defenses, particularly glutathione, via the **Nrf2** pathway, among others. This balances oxidation and reduction and reduces **(NF)-κB** activation, an inflammatory marker, which, when elevated, can lead to unhealthy cell growth. **Many uninformed**

researchers in the past have tried to make the case that antioxidants inhibit cytotoxic allopathic treatments for abnormal cells from working properly. However, this is simply a failure to understand the true role that antioxidants play and a reductionist mindset only focusing on the killing of abnormal cells without adequately understanding the complexity of the entire picture and phases of unhealthy cell growth and without considering the side effects such cytotoxic allopathic treatments have on healthy cells. A systematic review from 2016 that included 49 reports concluded that there is no evidence of antioxidant supplementation causing harm alongside abnormal cell therapy, except in the case of smokers undergoing radiotherapy, yet the review also mentioned a study that found that supplementing with antioxidants slightly increased survival in those undergoing chemotherapy, (Yasueda, Urushima, Ito et al.). Plus, these studies were primarily on isolate SUPPLEMENTS. Don't we all know by now that foods or food supplements are even better than isolates? In addition, plenty of studies have shown the ability of phytochemicals to act as "potent radiosensitizers" and enhance the efficacy of radiotherapy, while mitigating side effects, (Thyagarajan, Sahu et al.). See towards the bottom of the last page of these sheets for more info. Anyway, here are some "antioxidant" supplements with dual action for redox homeostasis: chlorogenic acid (green coffee bean), EGCG (green tea), catechin and epicatechin (cocoa or green tea), resveratrol, vitamin C, apigenin, luteolin, quercetin, curcumin, (andrographolide) andrographis, glutathione, ellagic acid (pomegranate), rosmarinic acid and carnosic acid (rosemary), COQ10, zurumbone (ginger), sulforaphane, curcumin. (Wang, Khor, Kong et al.), (Smith, Tran, Smith, McDonald...et al.), (Forman, Davies, Ursini et al.). **COX2** is an inflammatory enzyme also correlated with carcinogenesis, (Cerella, Sobolewski Dicato, Diederich et al.). **COX2 inhibitors/modulators:** astaxanthin, curcumin, resveratrol, EGCG, ferulic acid, beta carotene, quercetin, genistein (soy), omega 3s, (Desai, Prickril, Rasooly et al.), (Rao, Janakiram, Mohammed et al.). **5LOX** is another inflammatory enzyme overexpressed in abnormal cells. (Rao, Janakiram, Mohammed et al.) **5LOX inhibitors:** boswellia, omega 3s, curcumin, honey, *Terminalia chebula*, (Yadav, Prasad, Sung et al.), (Rao, Janakiram, Mohammed et al.). **Interleukin 1 and 2:** Interleukins are a group of cytokines that mediate communication between cells and regulate cell growth, immune responses, inflammation, and so on. Boosting Interleukin 1 may boost Interleukin 2 and strengthen the immune system's ability to knock out abnormal cells. At the same time, excessive interleukin 1 has been implicated in the aging process, destruction of cartilage, and inflammatory conditions. Chondroitin sulfate may help to inhibit IL-1 from damaging cartilage. **Interleukin 1/2 boosters:** beta glucans (mushrooms, oats, nutritional yeast), chlorella, carnosine, spirulina, bromelain, black cumin, astragalus.

2. Anaerobic glycolysis and aerobic glycolysis: Abnormal cells rely on either anaerobic glycolysis of sugar to run their metabolism and/or aerobic glycolysis (the Warburg effect). These processes can also be referred to as fermentation and the byproduct is lactate instead of CO_2. Normal, healthy cells rely on aerobic respiration, or, require oxygen to run their metabolism and function via mitochondrial **oxidative phosphorylation (OXPHOS)**, with CO_2 as a byproduct. If cells and mitochondria become damaged by ROS and starved of oxygen (hypoxic stress) and do not die, they may transform into abnormal cells and generate more ROS and create a more acidic environment in the body, (Vigani et al.), (Seyfried et al.). Hypoxia induces HIF-1α activation and shifts cells towards a glycolytic phenotype, (Maxwell, Pugh, Ratcliffe et al.). Iron is the main regulating nutrient of oxygen in the body. Both iron deficiency and iron overload may cause abnormal cells, (Fischer-Fodor, Miklasova, Berindan-Neagoe...et al.). Balancing iron levels may be important to maintain healthy cell growth, (Fischer-Fodor, Miklasova, Berindan-Neagoe...et al.). **Glycolysis regulators:** neoalbaconol from sheep polypore mushrooms, prosapogenin A from *Veratrum*, Epigallocatechin from *Spatholobus suberectus*, fisetin, myricetin, quercetin, apigenin, genistein (soy), cyanidin, daidzein (soy), hesperedin, naringenin, catechin, and carnosine, (Zhong, Qiang, Tan...et al.), (Gao, Chen et al.). **OXPHOS regulators:**

Chrysophanol, Shikonin, berberine, (Zhong, Qiang, Tan...et al.). **Hypoxia regulators:** papaya leaves, vitamin C (Zhong, Qiang, Tan...et al.). Metabolic nutrients and oxygenators may be needed prior to the formation of abnormal cells, however, some of the research on some of these nutrients is controversial once abnormal cells have already formed. Chlorophyll is an exception to that rule, however, I would say. **Metabolic nutrients:** carnitine, COQ10, ribose, creatine, alpha lipoic acid, chromium, iron bound with lactoferrin (to avoid the potential for iron to generate too many of its own ROS), PQQ, malic acid, citric acid, b-vitamins. **Oxygenators:** iron bound with lactoferrin, chlorophyll, chlorella, Dr. Chi Oxypower, carnitine, rhodiola, cordyceps.

3. Abnormal stem cells: The generation of abnormal stem cells may occur next. Abnormal stem cells are notoriously resistant to pharmaceutical drugs, (Taylor, Jabbarzadeh et al.). **Abnormal stem cell fighters:** resveratrol, curcumin (turmeric), quercetin, berberine (goldenseal), piperine (black pepper), capsaicin (cayenne), and vitamin A, (Taylor, Jabbarzadeh et al.).

4. Angiogenesis: Angiogenesis is new blood vessel growth. It is an undesirable process in the case of unhealthy cell growth because, the more blood delivered to these unhealthy cells, the more they can grow. **Tumor Necrosis Factor Alpha** is anti-angiogenic, meaning it reduces new blood vessel formation, thereby reducing blood supply to tumors. Boosting TNF-A short term may have anti-tumor effects, (Horssen, Hagen, Eggermont et al.). It should not be increased long term, however, as it is inflammatory. **Supplements that may increase Tumor Necrosis Factor Alpha:** Echinacea purpurea, mushrooms, bromelain, papain, pancreatin, SOD (increases effectiveness and inhibits toxicity of TNF), algae, seaweed, black cumin, Chinese ginseng, astragalus. Ginkgo, dandelion, UV-A exposure, and cat's claw may decrease the production of TNF-A. **Other anti-angiogenic supplements:** turmeric, grape seed extract, sea cucumber extract, licorice, lavender, ginseng, vitamin E, tocotrienols, red propolis, (Wargasetia, Widodo, et al.), (Morbidelli, Donnini, Turzuoli et al.), (Schindler, Mentlein et al.), (Nakagawa, Shibata, Yamashita et al.). **Foods that may be anti-angiogenic:** green tea, berries, citrus fruits, apples, pineapple, cherries, red grapes, bok choy, kale, soy, artichokes, nutmeg, pumpkin, parsley, garlic, tomatoes, dark chocolate, maitake mushrooms, ginger, pomegranate, cinnamon, (Angiogenesis Foundation), (Morbidelli, Donnini, Turzuoli et al.).

5. Survival: abnormal cells are able to survive by the alteration of the p53 gene, thereby preventing the induction of apoptosis. **Apoptosis** is programmed cell death or cell suicide. It is a natural process wherein mutated or unhealthy cells kill themselves. It is necessary to augment this process to reduce the survival of unhealthy cells. **Apoptosis inducers:** a huge variety of flavonoids such as fisetin, genistein (soy), daidzein (soy), acacetin, tangertin (tangerines), kaempferol, quercetin, pelargonidin, wogonin, delphinidin (maqui), etc., ellagic acid (pomegranate), curcumin, EGCG (green tea), lycopene (cooked tomatoes), pycnogenol, allicin (garlic), gingerol, gallic acid, baicelin (Chinese skullcap), vitamin C and D, saw palmetto, ashwagandha, silymarin, sea cucumber extract, tocotrienols, xanthohumol (hops), indole 3 carbonol, black seed, resveratrol, propolis, vitamin K3, and berberine via AP-1, (Abotaleb, Samuel, Varghese...et al.), (Wargasetia, Widodo, et al.), (Pratheeshkumar, Sreekala, Zhang, Budhraja...et al.), (Zhou, Zheng, Li...et al.), (Suresh, Raghu, Karunagaran et al.), (Agbarya, Ruimi, Epelbaum...et al.), (Wang, Khor, Shu, Su...et al.), (Mollazadeh, Afshari, Hosseinzadeh et al.),(Gupta, Kim, Aggarwal et al.). **Glycolysis:** Sugar feeds abnormal cells, allowing for their survival. Abnormal cells breakdown sugar to create energy. See the list of glycolysis inhibitors/regulators above and do not consume excessive refined sugars and refined carbohydrates. **Senescence:** In some circumstances, if there is less severe damage to DNA within a cell, then the cell may undergo senescence instead of apoptosis. Senescence is a state of permanent cell cycle arrest so that the cell can no longer replicate, yet the cell does not die. It is a mechanism enacted by the body to prevent the replication of aberrant cells, yet at the same time, the compounds secreted by senescent cells can contribute to aging and create a microenvironment conducive to the formation of aberrant cells. Therefore, the chronic buildup of excessive senescent cells is undesirable. As usual, the body is a paradox. Nrf2 and the p53/p21 and p16INK4a/pRB pathways regulate senescence, among other pathways. It is the job of one's immune system to destroy senescent cells, specifically, natural killer cells, macrophages, and T cells are tasked. Obviously, a weakened immune system may allow for the buildup of senescent cells. See the sheet entitled "Healthy Cell Growth – 5 Categories" for how to supercharge your immune system. **Telomerase and Immortalization:** Telomerase is expressed in roughly 90% of malignant cells and neoplasms, whereas healthy cells do not contain detectable levels of telomerase, (Eitsuka, Nakagawa, Kato...et al.). Telomerase is an enzyme that can lengthen telomeres on unhealthy cells and allow them to become immortal. Abnormal cells actually more commonly exhibit short telomeres, so the lengthening of them by telomerase ends up making their length about average. Telomeres are the ends of DNA strands, which, naturally, as a cell ages, get shorter, eventually leading to death of the cell. However, as usual, telomerase plays different roles in healthy cells versus unhealthy cells. Telomerase is good for healthy cells that are simply aging as it makes them even healthier and resist the aging process. Telomerase is controlled primarily by the transcription factor c-Myc and the catalytic protein subunit hTERT. Here is one **natural compound that inhibits telomerase activity in abnormal cells, yet does not inhibit it in healthy cells:** EGCG (green tea) (Naasani, Oh-hashi, Oh-hara...et al.). It is probably safe to assume that many of the other natural compounds studied to inhibit telomerase in abnormal cells do not inhibit it in healthy cells and rather play a role in telomerase homeostasis because natural dietary compounds are generally nontoxic to healthy cells, (Eitsuka, Nakagawa, Kato...et al.). Plus, a number of natural compounds have been shown to lengthen telomeres in aging, non-cancerous cells, (Tsoukalas, Fragkiadaki, Docea...et al.), (Tsoukalas, Fragkiadaki, Docea...et al.). However, I cannot research every single study on telomerase. **Here are some natural compounds that inhibit telomerase activity in abnormal cells. Whether they inhibit it in healthy cells, I do not know, but I highly doubt it, due to my arguments above:** retinol (vitamin A), curcumin, resveratrol, tocotrienols, pterostilbene (blueberries), indole 3 carbonol, diosgenin, gingerol, papaverine (poppy), butylidenephthalide (*Angelica sinensis*), crocin (saffron), dideoxypetrosynol A (marine sponge *Petrosia*), helenalin (*Arnica montana*), curcumin, glycoprotein LJPG (kombu), sylbinin (milk thistle), gallic acid (chamber bitter), ginenoside Rk1 (*Panax ginseng* (sun ginseng)), curcubitacins (snake gourd), boldine (boldo), gambogic acid (*Garcinia hurburyi*), sanguinarine (blood root), phenolic acids (*Cordyceps militaris*), (Eitsuka, Nakagawa, Kato...et al.), (Li, Chen, Yeh, Wang, Chen et al.), (Ganesan, Xu et al.).

6. Mitosis: Mitosis is cell division. It proceeds at a fast, uncontrolled rate in unhealthy cell growth. **Antimitotics:** withaferin A (Ashwagandha (not KSM-66)), pterocarpans, rough cocklebur, *Kalanchoe tubiflora*, maytansinoids (*Maytenus serrata, Maytenus ovatus*), *Cantharanthus* alkaloids, taxanes (European Yew and Pacific Yew), combrestatin A-4 (*Combretum caffrum*), Piclitaxel, vinca alkaloids (periwinkle), epothilones (*Sorangium cellulosum*), colchicine (Autumn Croccus), etc. (Paier, Maranhão,I,II, Carneiro,I,III,IV...et al.), (Sánchez-Lamar, Piloto-Ferrer, Fiore...et al.), (Hsieh, Yang, Leu...et al.), (Nagle, Hur, Gray et al.), (Lichota, Gwozdzinski et al.).

7. Growth: excessive levels of certain growth factors may contribute to abnormal cell growth and proliferation especially at the G1/S1 boundary of the cell cycle. Excessive amounts of animal protein may increase growth factors such as IGF-1 (Taha, Koshiyama, Mandai et al.), (Levine, Suarez, Longo et al.) and the enzyme MFO which may activate carcinogens (Campbell et al.). **Growth factor reducers:** black cumin (FGF), Fritillaria thunbergii (IGF-1), garlic (thymidine, VEGF, FGF2), lycopene (IGF-1), quercetin (EGF, VEGF), parsley (VEGF), chili pepper (VEGF), curcumin (EGF,

VEGF, bFGF), green tea (VEGF), resveratrol (FGF, VEGF), soy (FGF2, VEGF), vanilla bean (HGF), cloves (VEGF), sulforaphane (PDGF, VEGF), (Gupta, Kim, Aggarwal et al.), (Wargovich, Morris, Weber et al.), (Agbarya, Ruimi, Epelbaum...et al.). **Cell cycle arrest at G1 – S1 phase transition:** Boswellia, berberine, capsaicin (cayenne), curcumin, genistein (soy), guggul, ginger, sulforaphane, (Gupta, Kim, Aggarwal et al.).

8. Metastasis and invasion: Metastasis is the spread of abnormal cells. It involves growth, adhesion via ICAM, migration, and proteolytic degradation of tissue barriers by increasing MMP. **Metastasis and invasion blockers:** vitamin D, aloe, diosmin, modified citrus pectin, B17, DHA, EPA, fucoidan, reishi. (Glinski, Raz et al.), (American Society for Investigative Pathology), (Zhang, Lv, Qu, Chen...et al.), (Martínez, Vicente, Yáñez...et al.), (Liczbiński, Bukowska et al.), (Sohretoglu, Huang et al.), (Iigo, Nakagawa, Ishikawa...et al.), (Hsu, Hwang et al.). **Migration inhibitors:** berberine, catechin (green tea), capsaicin (cayenne), lycopene, vanillin, butein, genistein (soy), (Gupta, Kim, Prasad, Aggarwal et al.). **Adhesion (ICAM) blockers:** allicin (raw garlic or enteric coated garlic), apigenin, crocetin, (saffron), genistein (soy), B17, (Gupta, Kim, Aggarwal et al.), (Gupta, Kim, Prasad, Aggarwal et al.), (Liczbiński, Bukowska et al.). **MMP inhibitors:** caffeic acid, carnosol (oregano), gingerol (ginger), celastrol (thunder god vine), piperine (black pepper), curcumin, crocetin, (Gupta, Kim, Prasad, Aggarwal et al.).

More info on popular natural products with anti-abnormal cell effects: graviola - apoptotic, antiproliferative, cytotoxicity, necrosis (Qazi, Siddiqui, Jahan), (Rady, Bloch, Chamcheu...et al.), **B17** - apoptosis, (Saleem, Asif, Asif...et al.), **grapeseed extract** - antiangiogenic, antimetastatic, apoptosis, growth factors, aromatase, growth, cytotoxicity, (Kaur, Agarwal, Agarwal...et al.), **IP6** - antiproliferative, antimetastatic, cell cycle arrest, enhance efficacy of chemo, (Vucenik, Shamsuddin et al.), **sea cucumber** - cytotoxicity, apoptosis, cell cycle arrest, growth, antiangiogenic, antimetastatic, inhibition of drug resistance, (Wargasetia, Widodo, et al.), **mushrooms** - growth inhibition, cytotoxicity, growth arrest, apoptosis, antiangiogenic, antiinvasive, antiproliferative, migration inhibition, immunostimulation, increase TH1, (Blagodatski, Yatsunskaya, Mikhailova...et al.), (Guggenheim, Wright, Zwickey).

Increase the effectiveness of cytotoxic allopathic treatments (chemo and radiotherapy) for abnormal cells, reduce their toxicity, and mitigate their side effects: mushrooms, (Blagodatski, Yatsunskaya, Mikhailova et al.), (Ayeka et al.), (Guggenheim, Wright, Zwickey), (Patel, Goyal et al.). **Increase the effectiveness of radiotherapy and reduce its toxicity:** genistein, daidzein, glycitein, resveratrol, piperine, hydroxychalcones, (Thyagarajan, Sahu et al.). **Reduce side effects of chemotherapy:** astragalus, panax ginseng, (Chen, May, Zhou...et al.). **Reduce side effects of radiation:** aloe, honey, calendula, (Aghamohamamdi, Hosseinimehr et al.). **Reduce toxicity of radiation and chemo:** grapeseed extract, bacopa, aloe, rhemannia, red ginseng, green tea, milk thistle, pomegranate, ashwagandha, pine bark, curcumin, astaxanthin, vitamin E, (Olaku, Ojukwu, Zia, White et al.), (Zhang, Wang, Jia, Kong et al.). **Reduce toxicity of chemotherapy:** glutathione, melatonin, vitamin A and E, NAC, selenium, l-carnitine, Co-Q10, ellagic acid, vitamin C and E with beta-carotene or selenium, vitamin D, b-complex, (Thyagarajan, Sahu et al.), (Singh, Bhori, Kasu...et al.). **Reduce toxicity of radiation:** curcumin, lycopene, glutamine, tocotrienol, milk thistle, rutin, (Hall, Rudrawar, Zunk...et al.)

There are so many pathways and markers that come into play in supporting healthy cell growth such as **STAT3, MAPKs, IL-6, PGE2, Protein Kinase C, mutagens/PAHs, oncogenes, mTOR, caspases, bcl-2,** etc etc. We cannot cover them all, plus, some of these are upstream or downstream from other pathways/markers already covered here. But, for good measure, **vitamin E** hits a lot of them, including oncogenes, PGE2, Protein Kinase C, and PAHs.

Available for download @ collingowcnc.wixsite.com/collingowcnc/articlesandprotocols

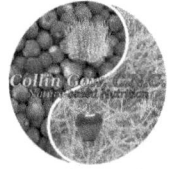

Healthy Cell Growth—5 Categories

Be sure to pick up the "Healthy Cell Growth – 8 Phases" sheet in addition to this sheet on the subject.

1. Remain alkaline: The only foods that are alkaline in nature are fruits and vegetables. Fats and millet can be neutral. Everything else is acidic. However, certain acidic things, such as certain amino acids, can play a role in balancing PH. Also, organic acids from sour foods such as citrus fruits, raspberries, green apples, etc. are important to run your metabolism. Organic acids from food sources in moderation are healthy and should generally not be completely avoided. When talking about getting alkaline, people are referring to having alkaline blood. Most of the rest of the body prefers to be slightly acidic, such as the stomach, the large intestine, the muscles, vacuoles within the cytoplasm of cells, and so on. When it comes to healthy cell growth, let's not complicate this. Here are some **alkalizers:** baking soda (sodium bicarbonate), calcium, Willard water, greens powders, fruits and veggies, bentonite clay.

2. Supercharge the immune system: In general, mushrooms are the strongest things in nature for the immune system. The strongest antiviral known is a mushroom (agarikon), we derive our antibiotics from mushrooms, and they are well documented to fight abnormal cells, mitigate the side effects of cytotoxic pharmaceutical treatments for abnormal cells, and may improve the effectiveness of such treatments, (Guggenheim, Wright, Zwickey et al.). The best thing about mushrooms is that they do not just indiscriminately "boost" the immune system, but, rather, they educate, modulate, and balance the immune system. They tell the body what to attack and what not to attack. **Mushrooms and other immunomodulators:** cordyceps, reishi, chaga, maitake, shiitake, agarikon, turkey tail, lion's mane, adaptogenic herbs, plant sterols, aged garlic extract, cat's claw, nutritional yeast, etc. **Other good immune system strengtheners and/or natural antimicrobials:** Artemisia annua (wormwood), andrographis, olive leaf, vitamin A, D, E, C, Selenium, Zinc, propolis, garlic with allicin, oregano oil, silver, licorice, lemon balm, goldenseal, echinacea, astragalus, etc.

3. Detoxify: The bottom line, with any particular ailment is, you are not healthy. Health comes down to two primary things: get A LOT of the good in and get the bad out. Sometimes, it's not the abnormal cells that kill a person, it's the detoxification pathways that are so overloaded, that organs begin to fail. Detox of the liver, lymphatic system, kidneys, blood, colon, and so on is paramount. **Detoxifiers:** Essiac tea, echinacea, dandelion, artichoke, yellow dock, burdock, red root, milk thistle, sulforaphane, glutathione, broccoli seed extract, mushrooms, parsley, cranberry, juniper, uva ursi, probiotics, psyllium, flax, chia, bentonite clay, etc.

4. Xenoestrogens: These usually come in the form of industrial chemicals that mimic estrogen and are endocrine disruptors. These can occur in herbicides, pesticides, other chemicals, plastics, unnatural cosmetics, carpet, organic and non-organic milk, animal products, non-organic foods, basically, anything that is not natural could potentially contain xenoestrogens. Try to eliminate as many unnatural things from your life as possible. **Xenoestrogen detoxifiers:** glutathione, TMG, methylcobalamin, MSM, raw cruciferous veggies, DIM, sulforaphane, NAC, calcium d-glucarate, indole 3 carbonol. Vitamin E may help to balance progesterone:estrogen ratio.

5. Organic, whole food, plant-based diet: There are 2 major options when it comes to a dietary approach to having healthy cells, either eating an organic, whole food, plant-based diet or keto diet. The idea behind the keto diet is that one starves the abnormal cells of their main fuel source, sugar, thus helping to kill them. However, the keto diet is not a healthy diet for the long term, in my opinion. First of all, it is an acidic diet, as ketones themselves are acidic. Diabetics seek to manage their blood sugar properly in order to avoid ketoacidosis, for instance. Ketoacidosis causes much harm to the body. Secondly, the keto diet, being higher in animal foods, is high in arachidonic acid, which is an inflammatory omega 6, so it is a more inflammatory diet. Thirdly, the diet is too narrow. Without supplementing it properly, a person will end up deficient in potassium (because fruit is not allowed and no, eating one or two avocados per day is not going to cut it), fiber, electrolytes in general, because they are needed to buffer the acidic nature of the diet, and many other nutrients. Also, excessive meat raises insulin and growth factors, which are not good for maintaining healthy cells. Not to mention the fact that most pathogens humans are exposed to from diet are zoonotic in origin (coming from animals). Lastly, most people will not be able to process and digest such a high fat diet properly because of a clogged up liver and gallbladder and they may exacerbate heart disease on such a diet, if not done properly. I said lastly, but one more thing, ketones are potent cross-linking agents too, acting like advanced glycation end products, which are harmful to the body. The whole food, plant-based approach is a healthier diet in my view, and, to me, no matter what the ailment is, the goal should always be to get healthy. Treating labeled conditions without supporting overall health doesn't work for serious issues. This being said, I'm not recommending doing large portions of fruit on a whole food, plant-based diet either, as abnormal cells rely on sugar as their fuel source (though potassium in fruit does help metabolize sugar anyway). See the two sheets on foods to eat and foods to avoid for healthy cell growth for more info.

Available for download @ collingowcnc.wixsite.com/collingowcnc/articlesandprotocols

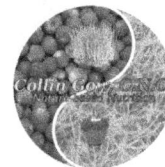

Healthy Cell Growth—Causes

Below is a list of factors associated with abnormal cell growth and some supplements and lifestyle changes that may target such factors. Be sure to pick up the other sheets on healthy cell growth for more info.

Infection (Masrour-Roudsari, Ebrahimpour et al.), (Faden et al.), (De Flora, La Maestra et al.): oregano oil, propolis, grapefruit seed extract, garlic, silver, *artemisia annua*, goldenseal, berberine.

Inflammation/oxidative stress (Coussens, Werb et al.), (Liu, Ren, Zhang…et al.): curcumin, boswellia, grapeseed extract, rosemary, ginger, garlic, lycopene, quercetin, andrographis, vitamin E, tocotrienols, resveratrol, green tea, reishi, cat's claw, omega 3s, glutathione, SOD, luteolin, apigenin, etc.

Weakened Immune system (Corthay et al.): Pre, pro, and postbiotics, mushrooms, andrographis, olive leaf, cat's claw, echinacea, garlic, vitamins A, E, D, C, minerals zinc and selenium, colostrum, shilajit, plant sterols, etc.

Mitochondrial/Metabolic conditions (Seyfried et al.): chromium, carnitine, coq10, pqq, alpha lipoic acid, iron bound with lactoferrin, ribose, b-vitamins, creatine, iodine, copper.

Improper cooking (John, Stern, Koo et al.), (Joshi, Kim, Stern et al.), (Anderson, Sinha, Kulldorff,…et al.): no grilling, barbequeing, baking, roasting, frying, sauteing, or other forms of dry heat cooking. Use wet heat cooking instead such as boiling, braising, poaching, steaming, stewing, etc. at low temperatures or don't cook the food at all (eat more raw foods).

Genetic defects (Campbell et al.): the field of epigenetics says that it is the environment in one's body surrounding the cell membranes that regulate the expression of genes. Therefore, diet and lifestyle probably play the biggest role in regulating genetic expression. See the healthy cell growth food sheets for more info.

Diet and Lifestyle (Gupta, Kim, Aggarwal et al.): Eat an organic, whole food, 51% raw, plant-based diet. See the healthy cell growth food sheets for more info. Exercise. Get outdoors in nature. De-stress. Do what you love. Sleep at least 8 hours. Engage with a community of friends. Have a positive mindset. Believe in something. Be kind. Breathe. Drink clean water. Read. Journal.

Environmental contaminants/pollutants (Koriech et al.): do not buy anything containing synthetic ingredients or chemicals. Buy all natural, organic cosmetics, toiletries, food, medicines, cleaning products, containers, clothing, furniture, paints, pots, pans, etc. Do not use plastic, pesticides, herbicides, or other chemicals. Replace carpet with a naturally finished wood flooring. Avoid tap water at all costs. These precautions should reduce exposure to PBDEs, PCBs, dioxins, phthalates, heavy metals, parabens, polysterene, alkylphenols, and other xenobiotics/xenoestrogens/endocrine disruptors/toxins. Glutathione, TMG, methylcobalamin, DIM, broccoli seed extract, sulforaphane, MSM, garlic, milk thistle, SAM(E), NAC, echinacea, yellow dock, burdock, artichoke, dandelion, choline, methionine, inositol, calcium D-glucarate, psyllium, charcoal, bentonite, cilantro, uva ursi, red clover, burdock, barberry, alpha lipoic acid, mushrooms, and many others may help to detoxify these harmful substances.

Radiation exposure (Shah, Sachs, Wilson et al.): minimize exposure to x-rays at doctor and dentist visits, flying on airplanes, cell phone, T.V., watch, fluorescent lighting, and computer use, and foods with the Radura symbol on them or a statement on them saying "treated with irradiation". One can also buy cell phone and laptop shields that minimize exposure.

Hormonal imbalances (Parkin et al.), (Sherbet et al.), (Travis, Key et al.): these come about from environmental contaminants/pollutants, medications, congenital mutations, deficiencies, lifestyle factors, and so on. Get your estrone, estriol, estradiol, progesterone, testosterone, dhea, cortisol, and pregnenalone levels checked.

High insulin (Thomas, Rome, Ujvari et al.), (Pustylnikov, Costabile, Beghi...et al.): Meat and processed foods/refined sugar can all raise insulin substantially. Abide by the diet recommendation above. See the foods to eat and foods to avoid sheets for more info.

High or Low cholesterol (Kitahara, González, Freedman...et al.): Check your cholesterol levels. Of course, the HDL and LDL ratio and the particle size of LDL are important to know as well. Amla, guggul, red yeast rice, berberine, citrus bergamot, turmeric, fiber, omega 3s, plant sterols, may assist with healthy cholesterol levels. For low cholesterol, eat more calories and 2 egg yolks per day.

Available for download @ collingowcnc.wixsite.com/collingowcnc/articlesandprotocols

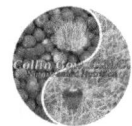

Healthy Cell Growth—Foods to Eat

It is believed that 90-95% of abnormal cell growth is caused by lifestyle factors and that 90% can be avoided by dietary changes, (Gupta, Kim, Aggarwal et al.). Below may be some healthy dietary approaches and healthy foods to add to your diet:

100% organic (Mie, Andersen, Grandjean et al.) (Baudry, Assmann, Touvier et al.)

51% raw (Link, Potter, et al.),

High Fiber (Donaldson et al.) (Pal, Banerjee, Ghosh et al.)

10 or more servings of vegetables per day (Donaldson et al.)

Either **Whole Food Plant Based, Vegetarian, Japanese, Mediterranean, Microbiota-regulating,** or **Keto** diet (Soldati, Renzo, De Lorenzo et al.), (Carruba, Cocciadiferro, Traina et al.), (Lanou, Svenson et al.), and especially**:**

Raw cruciferous vegetables such as kale, mustard greens, broccoli, broccoli sprouts, cauliflower, brussels sprouts, and cabbage (Carruba, Cocciadiferro, Traina et al.), (Donaldson et al.)

Mushrooms (all except portabello) (Shin, Kim, Lim, Kim, Sung, Lee, Ro et al.) (Zhang, Sugawara, Chen, Beelman, Tsuduki, Tomata, Matsuyama, Tsuji et al.)

Green tea (Carruba, Cocciadiferro, Traina et al.)

Organic soy (Carruba, Cocciadiferro, Traina et al.), (Takagi, Kano, Kaga et al.), (Applegate, Rowles, Erdman Jr. et al.)

Flax seeds and other seeds (Donaldson et al.) (Parikh, Maddaford, Pierce et al.) (De Silva, Alcorn et al.)

Brazil nuts and other nuts (Donaldson et al.) (Ip, Lisk et al.)

Herbs and spices (Kaefer, Milner et al.), (Butt, Naz, Qayyum et al.)

Raw onions and garlic (Pourzand, Tajaddini, Sanaat et al.)

Legumes (beans, peas, lentils, chickpeas, etc.) (Papandreou, Becerra-Tomás, Bulló...et al.) (Aune, De Stefani, Ronco, Boffetta...et al.)

Berries (Kristo, Klimis-Zacas, Sikalidis et al.), (Pan, Huang, Wang et al.)

Fermented Foods (Aragón, Perdigón, LeBlanc et al.), (Patra, Das, Shin et al.)

Available for download @ collingowcnc.wixsite.com/collingowcnc/articlesandprotocols

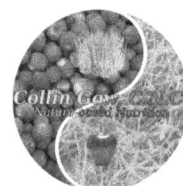

Healthy Cell Growth—Foods to Avoid

Excessive animal protein (Campbell et al.) (Taha, Koshiyama, Mandai et al.), (Levine, Suarez, Longo et al.)

Excessive animal foods (meat, eggs, milk, etc.) (Madigan, Karhu et al.)

Non-fermented Dairy (Lu, Chen, Wu et al.)

Alcohol (Koriech et al.), (Shield, Soerjomataram, Rehm et al.), (Vieira, Tobar, Thuler et al.)

Red and processed meat (Benarba et al.)

Grilled, barbequed, fried, and broiled meats (John, Stern, Koo et al.), (Joshi, Kim, Stern et al.), (Anderson, Sinha, Kulldorff,...et al.)

Excessive Sugar (Penson et al.)

Refined sugars (La Vecchia, Franceschi, Dolara, Bidoli, Barbone et al.)

Processed/Refined foods (Fiolet, Srour, Touvier et al.)

Non-organic foods (Baudry, Assmann, Touvier et al.)

Oils (Gerson et al.)

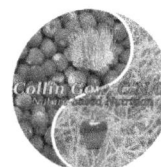

Healthy Cell Growth—Alternative Therapies

Vitamin C and K3 intravenous

Hyperbaric oxygen

Ozone

Hyperthermia

Molecular hydrogen therapy/Hydrogen PA

Coffee enemas

Hydrogen peroxide

B17 intravenous

Fasting/Caloric Restriction

Rife machine or similar device such as Zappers

Red light therapy

Bemer Therapy

Biomagnetic Cancer Therapy

Cryoablation

DMSO Potentiation Therapy (DPT)

Enzymatic Cancer Therapy

HALO Therapy

Immunotherapy

Anti-cancer vaccines

Mesenchymal

Cell therapy

Insulin Potentiation Therapy (IPT)

Intraperitoneal Perfusion Hyperthermia

Intravenous Curcumin

Intravenous GcMAF

Intravenous Solutions

DMSO

Customized IV Therapy

Laser Cancer Therapy

UVB

Peptide Treatment

Phenyl Butyrate IV

Radiofrequency Ablation

Salinomycin IV

Sonodynamic Therapy

Viral Anticancer Vaccine

LAK

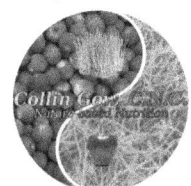

Immunity

Supplements

Daily use:

Mushrooms (maitake, shiitake, chaga, reishi, cordyceps, agarikon...) - immunomodulators (immune balancers), antitumor, antiinflammatory, antiviral. Agarikon is the strongest antiviral known.

Andrographis - antiinflammatory, antiviral, antimicrobial, antiprotozoa, antioxidant, blood sugar.

Astragalus - immunomodulator, anti-aging, adrenal health, kidney health, energy.

Echinacea (full spectrum extract) - boosts white blood cells including natural killer cells, moves and cleanses lymph. Good for pain in the neck under the jaw from swollen lymph nodes.

Olive leaf - contains oleuropein. Antifungal, antiviral, antibacterial, heart health, blood pressure, blood sugar. One of Abby's favorites. Slows viral shedding, budding, assembly, and replication.

Cat's Claw - antiinflammatory, immunodulator, antioxidant, antihypertensive, increases phagocytosis.

Licorice, marshmallow, aloe, slippery elm - immune cell communication, inhibit antigens of pathogens from attaching to cells, antiviral. Good for dry coughs and sore throats.

Aged garlic extract - immunomodulator, anticarcinogenic, Th1 immune responses, antioxidant.

Plant sterols - immunomodulators, do not take if you have very low cholesterol levels.

Elderberry - antiviral, febrifuge (lowers fever), decongestant. Good choice for kids because it tastes good.

Prebiotics, Probiotics, Postbiotics - 70% of the immune system is in the gut and there's more bacteria in your body than there are cells. Probiotics are foundational for a myriad of immune responses.

Shilajit/humic & fulvic acid - antiviral, immunomodulator, pro & anti-inflammatory, GABA mimetic.

Lysine - blocks the receptor sites where viruses try to secrete enzymes to spread through the body.

Vitamin A, C, E, D3, Zinc, Selenium - foundational vitamins and minerals which provide a host of immune benefits - NK cells, neutrophils, innate & adaptive immunity, macrophages, T & B cells, etc.

Colostrum or IGG - good source of antibodies. Antibodies tag pathogens so your immune system knows to destroy them. Important for innate immunity, GI health, and non-breastfed adults & children.

Temporary use:

Goldenseal - contains berberine. Antibacterial, anti-fungal, anti-protozoa, anti-viral, blood sugar, heart health, anti-inflammatory, anti-tumor. Good for pain in neck under the jaw line due to swollen lymph.

Grapefruit seed extract - antibacterial, antifungal, antiprotozoa, antiviral.

Silver - antiviral, antifungal, antibacterial, antiprotozoa. Good for ear, nose, throat, and eye infections.

Oregano oil - contains carvacrol. Antifungal, antibacterial, antiviral, antiprotozoa. Good for sinus congestion and respiratory infections in general.

Garlic containing allicin - antimicrobial, antifungal, antiviral, antiinflammatory.

Foods/Lifestyle

Limit processed foods and refined sugars. Limit high arginine foods (chocolate and nuts). Limit iron intake from foods and supplements. Limit dairy, meat, and other animal foods (organ meats are ok). Eat mushrooms, garlic, onions, ginger, peppers, fermented foods, manuka honey, citrus fruits, seaweed, and nutritional yeast. Nasal sprays, essential oils such as the four thieves remedy, ear oils, and hand washing are other precautionary measures one can take to reduce the spread of germs.

Available for download @ collingowcnc.wixsite.com/collingowcnc/articlesandprotocols

Menopause

Symptoms of menopause may include **hot flashes, breast tenderness, sleep disturbances, night sweats, irritability, mood swings, loss of libido, brain fog, vaginal dryness, painful intercourse, and more**. Perimenopause can begin as early as 35. Menopause may begin around age 40 – 58. During menopause the ovaries shut down and the adrenal glands must take over producing testosterone, estrogen, and progesterone. One usually needs to increase the good types of all of these hormones when in menopause.

1. Detox Harmful Estrogens and/or Block Aromatase

Calcium D-glucarate, DIM, Patented Glutathione, MSM, and TMG may assist with the detoxification of harmful industrial chemical estrogens from the body called "xenoestrogens" which activate unhealthy estrogen receptors (Erα). (Kelp or iodine should be taken when consuming DIM). **Dr. Chi Myomin, Chrysin, Pomegranate, Grapeseed, and Button Mushrooms** block aromatase. Aromatase converts testosterone into bad estrogens.

2. Add In Healthy Estrogens

Red raspberry leaf, licorice, black cohosh, red clover, sage, siberian rhubarb, and primrose oil contain natural phytoestrogens (plant estrogens) which bind to and activate healthy estrogen receptors (ERβ), allowing the modulation of estrogen levels and bringing them into a healthy balance. **Primrose oil** is also good for **vaginal dryness**. **Red raspberry** is a good choice for hot flashes, being both bitter and cooling and a phytoestrogen, but all of these herbs may be of assistance.

3. Raise Progesterone

Chaste tree increases leutenizing hormone which increases progesterone production. **Maca, Wild Yam,** and **Thyme** also raise Progesterone. Progesterone is required in 200x the level as estrogen by the body. Raising progesterone may help with sleep disturbances due to its modulation of GABA receptors.

4. Reduce Stress Hormones

Ashwagandha, Schizandra, Rhodiola, Holy basil, Reishi, Cordyceps, Maca, etc. are adaptogenic herbs that may lower stress hormones. Stress hormones compete with sex hormones and deplete them.

5. Take Actual Hormones If All Else Fails

Pregnenolone, DHEA, Progesterone, Estrogen in the form of Estriol, **and Testosterone** may all be taken in either pill or cream form. Be sure to take periodic breaks/cycle them.

Eat 25% of your caloric intake from fat. Healthy fats such as nuts and seeds, avocados, coconut butter, almond butter, hemp milk, organic, pasture raised hard-boiled egg yolks, small amounts of whole milk dairy such as: whole plain goat yogurt, whole goat cheese, and/or organic, grass fed, pasture raised A2 butter/cream, fatty fish with skin, coconut oil, olive oil (whole olives are too salty), hemp oil, fish oil, etc.

Consume seaweed, flax seeds, garbanzo beans, sesame seeds, parsley, organic tempeh, and organic miso for healthy phytoestrogens that activate ERβ. Eat at least one of these foods per day.

Available for download @ collingowcnc.wixsite.com/collingowcnc/articlesandprotocols

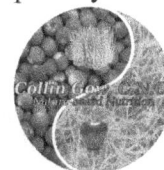

Sleep

A restful sleep of at least 8 hours or more per night is necessary to repair, recharge, detoxify, and recover from the daily grind. Insufficient sleep increases cortisol levels, pain, insulin resistance, hunger hormones, and psychological stress. **Among all primates, humans sleep the least**. This is a problem.

Lemon balm increases choline in the brain, which activates the parasympathetic nervous system, allowing you to relax. It's also antiviral. Viruses overstimulate the nervous system via the N-methyl-D-aspartate receptors. **St. John's Wort** is another calming, antiviral herb (do not take if on SSRI or SNRI antidepressant). **Skullcap, wild oats milky seed, poppy, valerian, and chamomile** are good nervine/antispasmodic/calmative/sedative herbs. **Ashwagandha** may help to balance stress hormones, mimic the effects of GABA, and help with **staying asleep**. **SAM(E)** helps metabolizes adrenaline.

GABA inhibits the neurons from over-firing, helping to quiet a racing mind from overthinking. Can use if you wake up in the middle of the night to get back to sleep (a snack may also help). **Passionflower** is the highest source of GABA in nature. Do not take GABA if on a benzodiazepine or Xanax.

Tryptophan converts into **5-HTP**, which converts into serotonin, then into melatonin (a sleep hormone). Serotonin regulates mood, appetite, sleep, and G.I. motility. (do not take if on SSRI or SNRI antidepressant)

Melatonin is a sleep hormone with antioxidant, antiinflammatory, antitumor, and cardioprotective effects. It may also slow cognitive decline, protect the macula of the eyes, and be beneficial for tinnitus sufferers. The human body does not usually naturally produce more than .3 mg of melatonin at night.

Magnesium is an essential macromineral and is involved in 300 different enzyme reactions in the body. 60-80% of the population is deficient in magnesium. It aids in relaxing the nerves and muscles and may reduce stress and tension. **Chloride** is necessary to make the enzyme that converts glutamine into GABA. **Zinc** is involved in 200 different enzymes in the body. It is essential for insulin to function properly, is a cofactor for the production of GABA, and may help with hyperactivity. High blood sugar may cause restlessness and an overactive mind. **Chromium** assists with the metabolism of sugar in the body, which may also support a peaceful sleep.

B6 and Iodine – B6 is necessary in the conversion of amino acids and may help with dream recall, while iodine helps to detoxify the pineal gland, which produces melatonin, allowing for more vivid dreams and deeper sleep. Do not take iodine at night, however. Take during the day.

Quercetin reduces histamine. Histamine acts as an excitatory neurotransmitter in the nervous system.

Dim lights 1 hour before bedtime (this includes the brightness on your phone!) to increase melatonin production. **Use a blue light filter** or buy blue light filtering glasses. Try **lavender oil** mixed with a carrier oil and rubbed on the feet. **Consume pistachios 30 minutes before bed** as they are the highest food source of melatonin in nature (much higher than cherries and lower in sugar). **Poppy seeds** are also good. **1 Tablespoon of coconut oil on toast** may help with **staying asleep**. **No high sugar, high potassium, high calcium, high protein, or allergenic foods late at night** (E.g. no refined carbs, cookies, ice cream, cakes, bananas, fruits, dairy, protein shakes, protein bars, meat, peanuts, corn, soy, wheat, or eggs within 1 hour of bedtime)

Available for download @ https://collingowcnc.wixsite.com/collingowcnc/articlesandprotocols

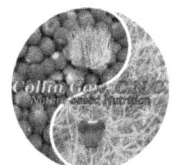

Testosterone

A higher testosterone level may improve mood, energy, sex drive, concentration, circulation, muscle strength, blood sugar, and hair growth among other benefits.

SUPPLEMENTS:
Nettles reduces sex hormone binding globulin allowing for higher Free Testosterone.

Pomegranate, Chrysin with Bioperine, Passionflower, Grapeseed, Dr. Chi Myomin, and Zyflammend Prostate inhibit aromatase. Aromatase converts testosterone into estrogen. Inhibiting aromatase may allow for higher T levels.

Adaptogenic herbs/supplements such as **Ashwagandha, Rhodiola, Schizandra, Holy Basil, Relora, Maca, Cordyceps**, and others reduce cortisol levels. Cortisol competes with testosterone.

Zinc is important for the health of the testes, sperm production, intensifies orgasm, and reduces 5-alpha-reductase. 5AR causes testosterone to convert into DHT which can clog hair follicles, causing hair loss.

Saw palmetto and **Beta-Sitosterol** reduce 5-alpha-reductase.

DIM, Broccoli seed extract, and Calcium D-glucarate help to detoxify xenoestrogens. These are toxic, cancer causing, industrial chemical estrogens that are rampant in the environment and they reduce free testosterone levels.

Tribulus (may increase the conversion of androstenedione into testosterone), **Tongkat Ali, Boron, Vitamin D3, Horny Goat Weed,** and **Fenugreek** (saponins stimulate the release of leutenizing hormone which stimulates the production of testosterone) are other good additions for low T.

Pregnenalone, DHEA, or Testosterone Creams may be used if actual hormones are needed. Be sure to take periodic breaks and cycle anything with actual hormones in it.

FOOD/LIFESTYLE:
Eat 25% of your caloric intake from fat. Choose healthy fats such as nuts and seeds, avocados, coconut butter, almond butter, hemp milk, organic, pasture raised hard-boiled egg yolks, small amounts of whole milk dairy such as: whole plain goat yogurt, whole goat cheese, and/or organic, grass fed, pasture raised A2 butter/cream, fatty fish with skin, coconut oil, olive oil (whole olives are too salty), hemp oil, fish oil, etc. Cholesterol and fat are necessary backbones to produce testosterone.
Eat organic.
Eat oysters, pumpkin seeds, raw cruciferous veggies, pomegranate kernels, and white button mushrooms.
Use less plastic, especially no acidic foods in plastic or microwaving in plastic or drinking out of plastic bottles.
Use all natural cosmetics, shampoos, soaps, and other body care products.

Download @ https://collingowcnc.wixsite.com/collingowcnc/articlesandprotocols

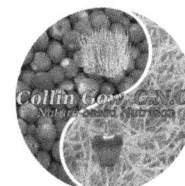

Thyroid

I often make the assumption that if a person lives in America, they are exposed to **municipal tap water**, and they do not consume seaweed on a daily basis, then they may have a thyroid problem, regardless of what blood tests may say. However, it's always good to get tests to confirm. The only significant source of **iodine** in the diet (the main nutrient the thyroid needs) is from seaweed. And very few Americans eat it. Meanwhile, we are constantly exposed to toxins that inhibit thyroid function such as harmful forms of fluorine, bromine, and chlorine. An important step to improving the thyroid is removing as many sources of these toxic **halogens** from your diet, lifestyle, cosmetics, and toiletries as possible. The thyroid produces 3 primary hormones – **T4, T3, and Calcitonin**. These hormones assist in **regulating metabolism, body temperature, blood pressure, pulse, growth, hair growth, brain development** (iodine deficiency is the most common cause of mental retardation in third world countries), **calcium, bone metabolism, and energy**. A doctor may diagnose you as having hypothyroidism if your **TSH** level is high. However, it can be good to get a full thyroid panel consisting of **TSH, total T4, T3, Reverse T3, ATA, and TPO** to get a more complete picture of what's going on. A **nodule** or **goiter** is a sign that the thyroid is severely iodine deficient and in trouble. **Hashimoto's** disease is an autoimmune condition that damages the thyroid and usually involves hypothyroidism (underactive thyroid), but can sometimes cause hyperthyroidism (overactive thyroid). **Immunomodulating supplements, adaptogens, heavy metal cleansers, and/or antivirals** may be necessary for this issue. One may also need iodine and other thyroid boosters if Hashimoto's is causing underactive thyroid function. **Selenium** may be especially important for Hashimoto's whether underactive or overactive. **Symptoms of low thyroid functioning include:** thinning hair, fatigue, dry skin, weight gain, puffy face or neck, cold hands and feet, muscle weakness, depression, impaired memory, slowed heart rate, and heavy or irregular periods.

Iodine, selenium, and **tyrosine.** Iodine and tyrosine are present in actual thyroid hormones (T4 and T3). Selenium is necessary to create the enzyme that converts T4 (inactive thyroid hormone) into T3 (active thyroid hormone). **Zinc** may also help with the conversion of T4 into T3. **Iron** helps with thyroid peroxidase production, assisting in creating thyroid hormones. **Copper** supports the hypothalamus' ability to regulate thyroid hormones. **Between 1,000 and 3,000mcg of iodine per day is a therapeutic dose.** Many people will cite that the Japanese get an average of 12.5mg of iodine from their diet on a daily basis, however, food sources of iodine are different than supplemental forms and taking that much iodine, especially without easing into it, may cause side effects. Iodine is an acidic, pro-oxidant mineral, and too much can actually cause hypothyroidism temporarily.

Guggul may increase iodine uptake by the thyroid and enhance the activities of thyroid peroxidase. **Hops** may stimulate iodine uptake by the thyroid and modulate hepatic expression of genes involved in thyroid hormone distribution and metabolism. **Coleus Forskholii** may activate cyclic AMP in the thyroid, potentiating the effect of TSH and increasing thyroid hormone secretion. The effect may be enhanced by calcium. **Thyroid glandulars** may provide a boost for the thyroid. New Zealand or Argentinian sourced is good.

Eat **Seaweed** and **Brazil nuts**. Get a **shower filter** and bathtub filter if you take baths. **Do not cook with non-stick pans**, choose stainless steel, cast iron, copper, or ceramic. **Wear gloves if you do dishes by hand. Do not swim in chlorinated swimming pools. Do not buy breads or juices from regular supermarkets** as they are often brominated. **Do not use fluoride containing toothpaste. Never drink tap water** that is not filtered. **Do not buy fluoridated baby water. If you eat pasta, only buy "artisanal pasta"** that uses bronze dye extruders (often imported from Italy).

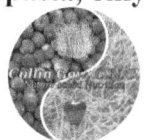

Thyroid 2

Hyperthyroidism (overactive thyroid) affects 1% of the population and is usually caused by **Grave's Disease**. Grave's disease is an autoimmune condition in which antibodies are produced that bind to TSH receptors in the thyroid, causing excessive thyroid hormone production and increased metabolism. **Grave's disease may be caused by toxic multinodular goitre or a toxic solitary nodule**. Grave's and Hashimoto's may be two different presentations of the same disease (Selenkow et al.). **It's important to realize that an overactive thyroid does not mean that you have an exceptionally well-functioning thyroid. On the contrary, thyroid gland inflammation and enlargement is occurring because the thyroid is not healthy.** It would make sense that the body would attempt to enlarge an organ's size to compensate for weak functioning of that gland, because it is unhealthy. So, I believe it to be the case that an overactive thyroid is usually one of the last stages in the same disease process that originally began as an underactive thyroid. **The main nutrient the thyroid needs to be healthy is iodine.** The goal, regardless of the thyroid issue, is to get the thyroid healthy. It is therefore my opinion that one needs iodine to improve thyroid health, whether the thyroid is overactive or underactive and iodine deficiency can cause both hypo- or hyperthyroidism (Zhongguo et al., Bülow et al.). **Tests: TSH, total T4, T3, Reverse T3, ATA, and TPO.** Low TSH and normal T4 and T3 may indicate hyperthyroidism. **Symptoms of hyperthyroidism:** hair loss, fatigue, ADHD, insomnia, heart palpitations or rapid heartbeat, elevated blood pressure, heat intolerance, irritability, nervousness, shortness of breath, tremors, muscle weakness, weight loss, bulging eyes, increase or decrease in appetite, sweating, elevated blood sugar, osteoporosis, anxiety, and brittle, shiny nails. Hyperthyroidism may increase the risk of Alzheimer's disease as well. Those with hyperthyroidism can experience **"thyroid storm"**. **If experiencing thyroid storm** (if heart rate, blood pressure, and body temperature soar to dangerously high levels) **seek immediate medical attention, as this can be life-threatening.**

Bugleweed is recommended in Ayurvedic Medicine for hyperthyroidism. Nervines such as **passionflower** and **lemon balm** may calm the nervous system and help with the symptoms caused by an overactive thyroid. Hyperthyroid patients have lower levels of **beta-carotene** (Aktuna et al.). **Vitamin A** deficiency has been linked with hyperthyroidism (El-Eshmawy et al.). 10,000 IU of vitamin A is the tolerable upper intake level for vitamin A. This is the highest dose an average adult could do every day forever with no problem, according to the government. Those with an overactive thyroid are at an increased risk of **carnitine** deficiency. Furthermore, **carnitine** may inhibit thyroid hormone entry into the nucleus of hepatocytes, neurons, and fibroblasts and may help with overactive thyroid symptoms, including the muscle weakness associated with it. (Benvenga et al., Sinclair et al.). **Quercetin** down regulates the expression of thyroid genes and inhibits thyroid function (Giuliani et al.). **Selenium** may benefit those with an overactive thyroid (Dharmasena et al.). 4 Brazil nuts per day may be a good selenium substitute. Overactive thyroid may be caused by **magnesium** deficiency. I believe **150mcg – 300mcg of iodine** is necessary for an overactive thyroid.

Eat **raw cruciferous vegetables** such as broccoli, kale, mustard greens, cabbage, cauliflower, Brussels sprouts, and broccoli sprouts **with dulse sprinkled on top. Eat orange, yellow, and red foods for vitamin A content**. The thyroid requires more vitamin A than any organ. **Eat lysine rich foods** such as pears **and iron rich foods** such as kale, spinach, beets, beef, liver, egg yolks, pumpkin seeds, molasses, cumin, parsley, etc. to assist with carnitine production in the body. **Millet** has antithyroid effects through the inhibition of TPO (Gaitan et al.). Get a **shower filter** and bathtub filter if you take baths. **Wear gloves if you do dishes by hand. Do not swim in chlorinated swimming pools. Do not cook with non-stick pans. Do not buy breads or juices from regular supermarkets. Do not use fluoride toothpaste. Never drink tap water that is not filtered. Do not buy fluoridated baby water.**

Foods

Superfoods

Raw cruciferous vegetables such as kale, mustard greens, broccoli, broccoli sprouts, cauliflower, brussels sprouts, and cabbage (contain sulforaphane, diindolylmethane, glutathione, good for Nrf2 activation, phase 2 liver detoxification, immune system, hormonal health – detoxify xenoestrogens)

Mushrooms (strongest things in nature for the immune system, immuno-modulating, good for hormonal health and nervous system health also, containing ergothionine, beta glucans, glyconutrients, aromatase inhibitors, and nerve growth factors)

Matcha green tea, black tea, black coffee (the highest source of antioxidants in the Standard American Diet. Life extension properties, high in polyphenols such as catechins and beneficial acids such as chlorogenic acid)

Flax seeds, chia seeds, savi seeds, hemp seeds, walnuts, wild caught salmon, and **sardines** (high in omega 3s, some contain moisturizing, lubricating, and hydrating GLA, Flax seeds rich in magnesium and contain lignans for hormonal balance, astaxanthin in salmon for eye, skin, joint, lung, and gut health, sardines high in calcium and COQ10)

Brazil nuts (richest source of selenium in nature and good for the immune system and thyroid)

Herbs and spices such as oregano, basil, cloves, cumin, garlic, cinnamon, cayenne, etc. (Herbs and spices are the 2nd highest on the nutrient density scale and the highest on the antioxidant scale)

Seaweed/algae such as dulse, laver, kelp, spirulina, etc. (highest sources of iodine and tyrosine in nature, good for the thyroid, energy, and metabolism, also contain lectin blocking mucilage (glyconutrients), good for gut and immune health, high in fiber, iron, and potassium)

Organ meats (most nutrient dense foods on the planet, high in zinc, iron, fat soluble vitamins, etc.)

Greens (high in blood building and detoxifying chlorophyll, folate, many other vitamins, minerals, and antioxidants)

Onions (high in sulfur and methionine, good for the immune system and detox)

Legumes (beans, peas, lentils, chickpeas, etc.) (high in iron, copper, manganese, fiber, and protein, important predictor of longevity, but also high in lectins)

Berries (high in antioxidant anthocyanins plus delphinidin in maqui berries and pterostilbene in blueberries, good for blood sugar, brain, blood vessels, and eyes)

Citrus fruits (high in organic acids, electrolytes, flavonoids, vitamin C, good for metabolism, energy, and hydration)

Fermented foods such as tempeh, miso, natto, umeboshi plums, kombucha, kimchi, sauerkraut, goat kefir, goat cheese, plain goat yogurt, etc. (pre, pro, and postbiotics, good for colon health, immune health, and metabolism, dairy sourced fermented foods high in calcium, good for bones and may help with maintenance of healthy blood pressure, soy sourced fermented foods good for bones and estrogen balance, high in isoflavones, daidzein, and genistein)

Bee products (contains terpenes, hormones, b-vitamins, vitamin b5, amino acids, silica, probiotics, go for immune system, bee pollen for allergies, royal jelly for stress – highest source of vitamin B5 in nature, propolis antimicrobial)

Salads (high in folate, enzymes, fiber, polyphenols, vitamins, minerals)

85% or higher dark chocolate (loaded with polyphenols, iron, magnesium, theobromine, and copper, boosts nitric oxide, good for circulation, good to assist healthy blood sugar levels, helps with energy)

Coconut and coconut water/products (abundance of medium chain triglycerides (MCTs) in coconut meat, oil, and butter, brain fuel, coconut water high in potassium and containing sodium, good electrolyte, good for hydration and energy)

Hot peppers (highest sources of vitamin C in nature, great for circulation, heart health, and blood sugar, vitamin C key for adrenal function also)

Aloe, slippery elm, licorice, marshmallow (major sources of mucilage, good for immune health, wound healing (often vulneraries in herbal medicine), gut health, lubrication, inflammation)

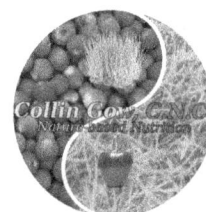

Healthy Carbohydrate Alternatives to Grains and Legumes

Semi-cooked sweet potatoes or yams

Semi-cooked purple potatoes

Semi-cooked white or red potatoes
(Even though these are nightshades, I still believe they are generally healthy as they are higher in nutrients and lower in lectins versus grains and lower in lectins and protease inhibitors versus legumes) (Latinos live longer than whites as a race because they eat legumes, however, legumes can cause unpleasant symptoms in some people with certain underlying ailments and a specific physiology, particularly in those with bloating and/or Type O blood)

Starchy vegetables such as carrots, beets, taro, yuca (cassava), daikon, cauliflower, etc.

Fruit

Buckwheat

Red or Black Quinoa

Millet (do not consume in excess if not supporting the thyroid with iodine or kelp)

If choosing any grains at all, then choose ancient, sprouted grains such as sprouted amaranth, spelt, einkorn, teff, kamut, farro, etc.

If choosing any legumes, then soak them overnight before cooking and eat with seaweed to block lectins and add carminative herbs such as cumin, ginger, fennel, caraway, or other spices such as turmeric, garlic, cayenne, etc. to aid digestion and reduce bloating.

Available for download @ collingowcnc.wixsite.com/collingowcnc/articlesandprotocols

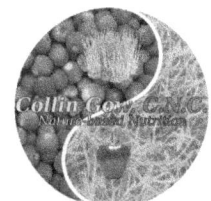

Weight Loss Foods

Fermented foods: kimchi, sauerkraut, umeboshi plums, tempeh, miso, kombucha, goat kefir, apple cider vinegar, etc.

Thyroid Foods: seaweed, Brazil nuts (4 per day)

B-vitamin rich foods: nutritional yeast, liver, kidneys, salmon, flax seeds, sesame seeds (high in fat, however), pistachios (high in fat, however), hot peppers.

Organic acid foods: sour foods such as citrus fruits, green apples, raspberries, golden berries, etc.

Pick low sugar fruits: green apples, greenish bananas, kiwis, berries

Xenoestrogen detoxifying foods: raw cruciferous vegetables such as kale, broccoli, Brussels sprouts, broccoli sprouts, cauliflower, cabbage, and mustard greens (add dulse flakes to them to support the thyroid).

Add spices to your diet such as cayenne, cinnamon, ginger, cumin, garlic, etc. as they are thermogenic and will raise metabolism.

Add Flax and Chia for fiber which will make you feel full without too many calories.

Drink green tea. It's about a 4% metabolism boost and healthy for you in many ways.

Eat balanced meals that contain fats, proteins, carbs, and fiber.

Reduce carbs slightly in these meals.

Choose healthy carbs such as fruits, veggies, sweet potatoes, purple potatoes, and beans.

Cook potatoes for less time so they are al dente (more firm) and eat the skin for the fiber content.

Try shirataki noodles (they are made from konjac root which is high fiber and contains no calories)

Avoid highly processed and refined foods, sweets, and junk food.

Available for download @ collingowcnc.wixsite.com/collingowcnc/articlesandprotocols

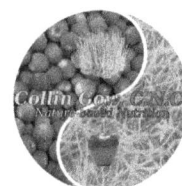

Briefings

Dear loyal clients, friends, and family,

This **flu season** has been an especially anxious and distressing one, with the **Coronavirus** threatening to become a pandemic. It's important not to panic, yet it is also important to take the necessary precautions to protect you and your loved ones. I have you and your family in my thoughts during this time and I am ready at the helm with natural remedies and immune system boosters to bolster your defenses. I thought I should prepare a short briefing on this topic and list my **top 10 recommended supplements** for your immune system.

What you need to know:

- Coronavirus was first detected in Wuhan City, Hubei Province, China and has now been detected in 57 locations internationally, including in the United States.
- It is a new form of the virus and it allegedly originated from bats.
- It causes respiratory disease and may cause death.
- It has been declared a public health emergency of international concern by the WHO.
- While cases have been detected in the U.S., according to the CDC, as of 2/28/20, the virus is NOT currently spreading in the community in the U.S.
- It spreads via animal to person and/or person to person via coughing, sneezing, close contact, etc. and can spread before a person has any symptoms.

My Top 10 Supplements

1. Astragalus
2. Silver
3. Oregano Oil
4. Olive Leaf
5. Vitamins A, C, D, E, Zinc, and Selenium
6. Elderberry
7. Andrographis
8. Mushrooms (Fomitopsis officinalis, Reishi, Shiitake, Maitake, Turkey Tail, Cordyceps, Chaga, etc.)
9. Echinacea
10. Berberine or Goldenseal

Other great options:

Pre, pro, and postbiotics, shilajit, colostrum or IGG, cat's claw, licorice or marshmallow, mucolase, oscillococcinum, garlic, grapefruit seed extract, lomatium, NAC, pleurisy, horehound, mullein, elecampane, yerba santa, thyme, eucalyptus, wild cherry bark, black seed oil, lysine, burdock.

What else?

Limit processed foods and refined sugars. Limit high arginine foods (chocolate and nuts). Limit iron intake from foods and supplements. Limit dairy, meat, and other animal foods. Eat mushrooms, garlic, onions, ginger, peppers, fermented foods, manuka honey, citrus fruits, seaweed, coconut, Brazil nuts, & nutritional yeast. Nasal sprays, essential oils, ear oils, and hand washing are also precautionary measures one can take which may possibly reduce the spread of germs. Should you come down with any virus this season, I recommend taking A LOT more than the bottle recommends just to be safe! Tripling, quadrupling, quintupling, or sextupling the recommended doses may be necessary! Ask your doctor or email me, however, and I/we will guide you on this. If you are a confirmed carrier of the Coronavirus, **seek immediate medical attention** and take measures so as not to spread the virus to others. In gratitude for your continued support of me, I am here to support you. Stay safe and be well.

Visit collingowcnc.wixsite.com/collingowcnc for more information.

These statements have not been evaluated by the FDA. This is not an attempt to treat, diagnose, prevent, or cure any disease or condition. Talk to your doctor before making any changes.

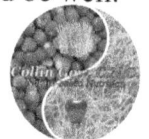

Dear citizens,

This **pandemic season** as of 2/29/20 has been an especially anxious and distressing one, as it usually is. The pattern continues, whether it's **swine flu, bird flu, SARS, MERS, West Nile, Ebola, Zika, Coronavirus**, or others, it seems that almost every year there's a new pathogen poised to reach pandemic proportions. Could any of these microbes have been perpetrated on the masses purposely to strike fear and obedience into them? It seems possible, if not likely, given such a predictable **pattern**. Out comes the virus, of which a patent on the vaccine for it was filed a year prior in secrecy, then it spreads, then ensues mass hysteria, it's all over every news channel, the experts warned of it a few months back, soon there's talk of a vaccine, then we are all saved by the mighty cow gods, then it mysteriously vanishes into thin air and we never think of it again (probably because there's another one next year to entertain us and draw our attention away from more important issues). The plan always seems to play out perfectly for the pharmaceutical companies and their pundits like precision clockwork. If indeed they are behind the farce, that is. The profits pour in while the poor press on, ignorant to the scheme of the billionaires. It matters little, however. You are likely not a billionaire and you must deal with the vermin that has been unleashed that threatens to vanquish you this very minute. It's important not to panic in this time of uncertainty and chaos, while the death toll allegedly rises, yet it is also important to take the necessary precautions to protect you and your loved ones. No, I don't mean using hand sanitizer and water and antibacterial soap. These are useful, sure, but I'm talking about real precautions. I do believe people are dying and I do believe the pathogen is real. So, I'm ready at the helm with natural remedies and immune system boosters to bolster your defenses. Your immune system is what you need most right now. So, here's a short briefing on this topic and my **top 10 natural antivirals/antimicrobials and immune system strengtheners**. Call it **Natural Pandemic Preparedness 101**, plus, some food recommendations to boot. I know, I know, I went way too far off the deep end on this one.

What to do when a pandemic strikes:
- Distrust the mainstream media (6 corporations own all of the mainstream media outlets)
- Do your own research
- Take it in perspective/proportion/context (realize that many more people die from the food they put in their mouths and from cancer and heart disease than any pathogen will probably ever cause. The media likes to blow things out of proportion to other important stories to push its agenda)
- Prepare yourself regardless (don't get so wrapped up in conspiracies about this year's pandemic that you don't take precautionary measures to protect and prepare yourself)
- Eat healthily
- Buy a face mask
- Stock up on natural medicines

My Top 10 Supplements
1. Astragalus
2. Silver
3. Oregano Oil
4. Olive Leaf
5. Vitamins A, C, D, E, Zinc, and Selenium
6. Elderberry
7. Andrographis
8. Mushrooms (Fomitopsis officinalis, Reishi, Shiitake, Maitake, Turkey Tail, Cordyceps, Chaga, etc.)
9. Echinacea

10. Berberine/Goldenseal

Other great options:

Pre, pro, and postbiotics, shilajit, colostrum or IGG, cat's claw, licorice or marshmallow, mucolase, oscillococcinum, garlic, grapefruit seed extract, lomatium, NAC, pleurisy, horehound, mullein, elecampane, yerba santa, thyme, eucalyptus, wild cherry bark, black seed oil, lysine, burdock.

What else?

Limit processed foods and refined sugars. Limit high arginine foods (chocolate and nuts). Limit iron intake from foods and supplements. Limit dairy, meat, and other animal foods. Eat mushrooms, garlic, onions, ginger, peppers, fermented foods, manuka honey, citrus fruits, seaweed, coconut, Brazil nuts, & nutritional yeast. Nasal sprays, essential oils, ear oils, and hand washing are also precautionary measures one can take which may possibly reduce the spread of germs. Should you come down with any virus this season, I recommend taking A LOT more than the bottle recommends just to be safe! Tripling, quadrupling, quintupling, or sextupling the recommended doses may be necessary! Ask your doctor or email me, however, and I/we will guide you on this. If you are a confirmed carrier of the Coronavirus, **seek immediate medical attention** and take measures so as not to spread the virus to others. In gratitude for your continued support of me, I am here to support you. Stay safe and be well.

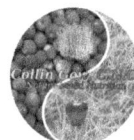

Practitioner Education Sheets

COVID-19 Epidemiology, Clinical Features, Hypothetical Regimens

by Collin Gow, C.N.C. (3/26/2020)

OVERVIEW

COVID-19 Fatality Rate by AGE:

*Death Rate = (number of deaths / number of cases) = **probability of dying if infected by the virus** (%). This probability differs depending on the age group. The percentages shown below do not have to add up to 100%, as they **do NOT represent share of deaths by age** group. Rather, it represents, for a person in a given age group, the **risk of dying** if infected with COVID-19.

AGE	DEATH RATE confirmed cases	DEATH RATE all cases
80+ years old	21.9%	14.8%
70-79 years old		8.0%
60-69 years old		3.6%
50-59 years old		1.3%
40-49 years old		0.4%
30-39 years old		0.2%
20-29 years old		0.2%
10-19 years old		0.2%
0-9 years old		no fatalities

*Death Rate = (number of deaths / number of cases) = **probability of dying if infected by the virus** (%).

Sources:
The Epidemiological Characteristics of an Outbreak of 2019 Novel Coronavirus Diseases (COVID-19) - China CCDC, February 17 2020

Report of the WHO-China Joint Mission on Coronavirus Disease 2019 (COVID-19) [Pdf] - World Health Organization, Feb. 28, 2020

Annual Risk Of Death During One's Lifetime

DISEASE AND ACCIDENTAL CAUSES OF DEATHS	ANNUAL DEATHS	DEATH RISK DURING ONE'S LIFETIME
Heart disease	652,486	1 in 5
Cancer	553,888	1 in 7
Stroke	150,074	1 in 24
Hospital Infections	99,000	1 in 38
Flu	59,664	1 in 63
Car accidents	44,757	1 in 84
Suicide	31,484	1 in 119
Accidental poisoning	19,456	1 in 193
MRSA (resistant bacteria)	19,000	1 in 197
Falls	17,229	1 in 218
Drowning	3,306	1 in 1,134
Bike accident	762	1 in 4,919
Air/space accident	742	1 in 5,051

Sources: All accidental death information from National Safety Council. Disease death information from Centers for Disease Control and Prevention. Shark fatality data provided by the International Shark Attack File.

Lifetime risk is calculated by dividing 2003 population (290,850,005) by the number of deaths, divided by 77.6, the life expectancy of a person born in 2003.

There's a .2% chance of dying from COVID-19 if you get it and if age 30-39. That's a 1 in 500 chance of dying from it if you get it. But that's probably the chance if you are under the care of a physician in an allopathic care setting, not if you're on natural meds. And the chance that you will get it is not 100% so it lowers the overall chance of dying from it to even less than .2%. But, let's just use the 1 in 500 number to give the benefit of the doubt that we are all going to get it and that we are all going to be treated allopathically. **A 1 in 500 chance of dying from corona is less of a chance than dying from falling, MRSA, accidental poisoning, suicide, car accidents, flu, hospital infections, stroke, cancer, and heart disease! If driving your car is more hazardous than corona, then why the big hubub about it?**

Symptoms: fever (most common symptom), cough, myalgia (muscle pain), fatigue, sore throat, mucus production, headache, trouble breathing, haemoptysis (coughing up blood), diarrhea.[1,2] **If symptoms become unbearable, seek immediate medical attention!**

Complications: pneumonia, lymphopenia (low lymphocyte count), leucopenia (low white blood cell count), cardiac injury, kidney injury, shock, secondary infection, respiratory distress, RNAaemia, prolonged prothrombin time (blood taking too long to clot), elevated D-Dimer (byproducts of fibrinolysis), hypoxia (low O_2).[1,2]

Other Clinical Features: high plasma concentrations of IL1B, IL1RA, IL7, IL8, IL9, IL10, basic FGF, GCSF, GMCSF, IFNγ, IP10, MCP1, MIP1A, MIP1B, PDGF, TNFα, and VEG upon admission.[1,2]

Conventional Treatment: antivirals (oseltamivir, etc.), antibiotics, corticosteroids, ventilation, nasal cannula, kidney transplant.[1,2]

Contraindications: ACE inhibitors & angiotensin receptor blocker meds may ↑ infect risk (Diaz et al.)

MUST HAVES

1. <u>Boost the immune system</u> – Pick 2 of the following and double the doses recommended on the bottles or do the max dose the bottle suggests: echinacea, astragalus, mushrooms, cat's claw, zinc (hydroxychloroquine works by pushing zinc into the cells), vitamin A, C, D3, E, selenium, colostrum, hGh, multivitamin. **Or pick 1 of the following and double the dose recommended on the bottle (but don't double the dose on the Source Naturals Wellness Formula):** Bluebonnet Wellness Support, Solaray Under the Weather Plus, Source Naturals Wellness Formula, Megafood Acute Defense, or Gaia Quick Defense. These formulas have many immune boosting ingredients in one product.

2. <u>Take antivirals studied against coronaviruses and/or HIV</u> (HIV-1-like inserts have been found in COVID-19)[3] **– Pick 1 of the following and quadruple the dose recommended on the bottle or pick 2 options and only double the dose on each bottle. Studied against coronaviruses:** red algae,[4] *Artemisia annua* (wormwood),[5] thyme,[6] oregano,[6] licorice,[7] nettle root,[8] peppermint,[6] horse chestnut,[9] or quercetin.[10] **Studied against HIV:** silver,[11] spirulina,[12] olive leaf,[13] *Artemisia annua*,[14] andrographis,[15] elderberry,[16] reishi.[17] **Other antivirals:** shilajit, goldenseal, agarikon, lysine. **I do not recommend high doses of garlic, only minimal to average doses** as it thins the blood too much for this particular issue.

3. <u>Reduce inflammation in the lungs</u> (Dr.s use corticosteroids as part of their treatment of COVID-19) **– Pick 1 of the following and double, triple, or quadruple the dose recommended on the bottle:** boswellia, black seed oil, ginger, turmeric, rosemary, bromelain, pancreatin, green tea, tart cherry, white willow, omega 3s, etc. **Or pick 1 of the following and double the dose recommended on the bottle:** New Chapter Zyflamend, Crystal Star Inflama Relief, Life Seasons Inflamma – X, Michael's Recovery Zymes or Wobenzym.

4. <u>Take a respiratory product</u> – Pick 1 of the following and use as directed, double, triple, or quadruple the dose recommended on the bottle: oregano oil, black seed oil, peppermint, eucalyptus, NAC, Terry Naturally Bronchial Clear Liquid, Dr. Chi Bamboo Extract, Old Indian Wild Cherry Bark syrup, Natural Factors Lung Bronchial and Sinus, Vitality Works Respir-Ease, (or herbs such as elecampane, lobelia, yerba santa, wild cherry bark, horehound, hyssop, mullein, marshmallow, thyme, etc. **And/or nebulize glutathione (Theranaturals brand) or silver or use a salt inhaler.**

5. <u>Boost oxygen levels without taking excessive iron (iron may feed pathogens)</u> (hypoxia is a complication of COVID-19 infection, hence ventilator and nasal cannula use in patients) **– Pick 1 of the following and double or triple the dose recommended on the bottle:** Chlorophyll, Chlorella, Chi Oxypower, Cordyceps, Rhodiola, Sun Warrior Liquid Light, Restore, CoQ10.

OPTIONAL

6. Take a febrifuge or antipyretic (fever reducer) (only if temperature goes above 104 degrees) - **Pick 1 of the following and double the dose recommended on the bottle:** ginger, peppermint, feverfew, cayenne, wormwood, black pepper, andrographis, yarrow, catnip, bergamot, white willow, Indian barberry, garlic, sage, holy basil, bitter melon, blood root, boneset, buchu, fenugreek, hops, horse chestnut, basically any spicy or bitter herb.

7. Boost vitamin K1 and calcium levels to assist with blood clotting (PTT and D-Dimer are elevated in COVID-19 patients) – **Follow the directions on the bottle:** drink a greens powder or eat lots of vegetables or take a minimum of 90mcg (female) or 120mcg (male) vitamin K1 per day either in or with a calcium supplement. New Chapter Bone Strength or Country Life Bone Solid are good choices. **These do not thicken the blood indiscriminately; they are only activated when there is an injury to the blood vessels.**

8. Strengthen capillaries (bleeding into the lungs may occur with acute COVID-19 infection) –**Follow the directions on the bottle or in some cases take less than recommended:** horse chestnut, butcher's broom, pine bark extract/pycnogenol, silica or Dr. Chi Bamboo Extract, collagen, Solaray Circulegs or Nature's Way Vein Support. **I do not recommend high doses of grapeseed extract in this instance, normal/average doses are ok.** Horse Chestnut best choice at it is also studied to be antiviral against coronaviruses.[9]

9. Keep the liver, lymphatic system, and kidneys clean (organ overload/failure may occur in COVID-19 infection) – **Pick 1 of the following and follow the suggested use on the bottle or take less:** burdock, yellow dock, dandelion, red clover, milk thistle, artichoke, red root, echinacea, chlorophyll, cornsilk, cleavers, buchu, parsley, juniper, NAC, glutathione, broccoli seed extract. **Or Pick 1 of the following formulas and use as suggested on the bottle or take less:** Lymphatonic by Herbs Etc, NOW Liver Renew, Gaia Liver Cleanse, Solaray Skin (a lymphatic/blood cleanser), Solaray Tetra Cleanse, Solaray Kidney.

Other Tips: Drink extra water to keep fever down, check temperature regularly, **wash hands, wear an N95 mask** if you must go out, **self-quarantine. Do go into stores. Have a friend or family member that hasn't been around you pick up your order curbside or buy online.**

Hypothetical Regimen 1:
1. **Source Naturals Wellness Formula (capsules)** – 2 caps, 3X/DAY with food
2. **Vibrant Health Gigartina** – 4 caps, 2X/DAY with food
3. **Terry Naturally Bosmed** – 2 softgels, 3X/DAY with food
4. **Old Indian Wild Cherry Bark Syrup** – 2 Tbsp, 2X/DAY
5. **World Organic Liquid Chlorophyll** – 1 Tbsp, 2X/DAY
6. **2 tea bags peppermint,** 2X/DAY only if temp. above 104 degrees
7. **New Chapter Bone Strength** – 1 slim tab, 3X/DAY with food
8. **Nature's Way Vein Support** – 1 capsule/DAY
9. **Liver/Lymphatic/Kidney cleanse may not be needed**

Hypothetical Regimen 2:
1. **Gaia Echinacea Supreme (Do not need to double the dose on this one as the bottle already recommends high doses)** – 4 caps, 4X/DAY (highest dose recommended on the bottle)
   NOW OptiZinc – 1 cap, 2X/DAY with food
2. **Natural Factors Oregano Oil softgels** – 1 softgel, 4X/DAY with food

3. **Crystal Star Inflama Relief** – 2 caps, 4X/DAY with food
4. **Country Life NAC 750mg** – 2 caps, 2X/DAY on empty stomach
5. **Chi Oxypower** – 3 caps, 2X/DAY with food
6. **Febrifuge/Antipyretic may not be needed**
7. **Solgar vitamin K1 100mcg** – 1 tab/DAY
8. **Country Life Pycnogenol 50mg** – 1/DAY with food
9. **Liver/Lymphatic/Kidney cleanse may not be needed**

Hypothetical Regimen 3:
1. **Megafood Women's One Daily Multi** – 1 tab, 2X/DAY
   Immune Tree Colostrum Powder – 1 tsp, 2X/DAY
2. **Sovereign Silver** – 1 tsp, 7X/DAY
3. **Solaray Ginger** – 2 caps, 3X/DAY with food
4. **Terry Naturally Bronchial Clear Liquid** – 2 tsp, 2X/DAY
5. **Health Force Chlorella** – 1 tsp, 2X/DAY
6. **Febrifuge/Antipyretic may not be needed**
7. **K1/Calcium may not be needed**
8. **Dr. Chi Bamboo Extract** – 2 caps, 3X/DAY with food
9. **Liver/Lymphatic/Kidney cleanse may not be needed**

Hypothetical Regimen 4:
1. **Bluebonnet Wellness Support** – 2 tabs, 2X/DAY with food
2. **Solaray Horse Chestnut Extract** – 1 cap, 2X/DAY
   Oregon's Wild Harvest Licorice – 3 caps, 2X/DAY
3. **Michael's Recovery Zymes** – 3 tabs, 2X/DAY on empty stomach
4. **Heritage Store Black Seed Oil** – 1 tsp, 2X/DAY with food
5. **Sun Warrior Liquid Light** – 1 capful, 2X/DAY with food
6. **Febrifuge/Antipyretic may not be needed**
7. **Bluebonnet Organic Greens Powder** – 1 scoop/DAY
8. **Capillary product may not be needed**
9. **Liver/Lymphatic/Kidney cleanse may not be needed**

Hypothetical Regimen 5:
1. **Host Defense Stamets 7 Powder** – 1 tsp, 2X/DAY with food
   Trace Mineral Research Power Pack Vitamin C packets – 1, 2X/DAY with food
2. **Gaia Olive Leaf Capsules** – 2 caps, 2X/DAY with food
   Gaia Elderberry Syrup – 2 tsp, 2X/DAY
3. **Terry Naturally Curamed 750** – 1 softgel, 3X/DAY with food
4. **Vitality Works Respir-Ease -** 1 dropperful, 3X/DAY
5. **Gaia Rhodiola Capsules** – 2 caps, 2X/DAY
6. **2 tea bags ginger,** 2X/DAY only if temp. above 104 degrees
7. **Country Life vitamin K1 100mcg** – 1 tab/DAY
8. **Harmonic Innerprizes Silica** – 1 capsule/DAY with food
9. **Herbs Etc Lymphatonic** – 1 dropperful/DAY
   Or World Organic Liquid Chlorophyll – 1 Tbsp/DAY

Hypothetical Regimen 6:
1. **Gaia Quick Defense** – 4 caps, 2X/DAY
2. **Sunfood Shilajit Powder** – 1/8th tsp, 2X/DAY with food

3. **New Chapter Zyflamend** – 2 caps, 2X/DAY with food
4. **Natural Factors Lung Bronchial and Sinus** – 2 tabs, 3X/DAY
5. **Host Defense Cordyceps Capsules** – 2 caps, 2X/DAY
6. **Febrifuge/Antipyretic may not be needed**
7. **Spirulina Powder** – 1 tsp/DAY
8. **Sun Warrior Collagen or Garden of Life Beauty Collagen** – 1 scoop/DAY
9. **Liver/Lymphatic/Kidney cleanse may not be needed**

Foods: Limit processed foods and refined sugars. Limit high arginine foods (chocolate and nuts). Limit iron intake from supplements. Limit dairy, meat, and other animal foods (organ meats are ok). Eat mushrooms, garlic, onions, ginger, peppers, fermented foods, manuka honey, citrus fruits, seaweed (especially dulse), brazil nuts, cooked oysters, pumpkin seeds, nutritional yeast, and puer or black tea.[18]

Available for download @ collingowcnc.wixsite.com/collingowcnc/articlesandprotocols

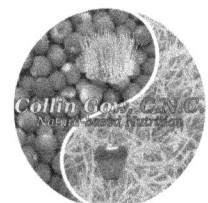

1 Huang, Chaolin & Wang, Yeming & Li, Xingwang & Ren, Lili & Zhao, Jianping & Hu, Yi & Zhang, Li & Fan, Guohui & Xu, Jiuyang & Gu, Xiaoying & Cheng, Zhenshun & Yu, Ting & Xia, Jiaan & Wei, Yuan & Wu, Wenjuan & Xie, Xuelei & Yin, Wen & Li, Hui & Liu, Min & Cao, Bin. (2020). Clinical features of patients infected with 2019 novel coronavirus in Wuhan, China. The Lancet. 395. 10.1016/S0140-6736(20)30183-5.

2 Cao, Min & Zhang, Dandan & Wang, Youhua & Lu, Yunfei & Zhu, Xiangdong & Li, Ying & Xue, Honghao & Lin, Yunxiao & Zhang, Min & Sun, Yiguo & Yang, Zongguo & Shi, Jia & Wang, Yi & Zhou, Chang & Dong, Yidan & Liu, Ping & Dudek, Steven & Xiao, Zhen & Lu, Hongzhou & Peng, Longping. (2020). Clinical Features of Patients Infected with the 2019 Novel Coronavirus (COVID-19) in Shanghai, China. 10.1101/2020.03.04.20030395.

3 Pradhan, Prashant & Pandey, Ashutosh & Mishra, Akhilesh & Gupta, Parul & Tripathi, Praveen & Menon, Manoj & Gomes, James & Perumal, Vivekanandan & Kundu, Bishwajit. (2020). Uncanny similarity of unique inserts in the 2019-nCoV spike protein to HIV-1 gp120 and Gag. 10.1101/2020.01.30.927871.

4 Lee, C. Griffithsin, a Highly Potent Broad-Spectrum Antiviral Lectin from Red Algae: From Discovery to Clinical Application. *Mar. Drugs* **2019**, *17*, 567.

5 Lin LT, Hsu WC, Lin CC. Antiviral natural products and herbal medicines. *J Tradit Complement Med*. 2014;4(1):24–35. doi:10.4103/2225-4110.124335

6 Lelešius, Raimundas & Karpovaitė, Agneta & Mickienė, Rūta & Drevinskas, Tomas & Tiso, Nicola & Ragazinskiene, Ona & Kubilienė, Loreta & Maruska, Audrius & Salomskas, Algirdas. (2019). In vitro antiviral activity of fifteen plant extracts against avian infectious bronchitis virus. BMC Veterinary Research. 15. 10.1186/s12917-019-1925-6.

7 Cinatl, Jindrich & Morgenstern, B & Bauer, G & Chandra, Prof & Rabenau, Holger & Doerr, Hans Wilhelm. (2003). Glycyrrhizin, an active component of liquorice roots, and replication of SARS-associated coronavirus. Lancet. 361. 2045-6. 10.1016/S0140-6736(03)13615-X.

8 van der Meer, Frank & de Haan, Cornelis & Schuurman, N & Haijema, Bert & Peumans, W & Damme, Els & Delputte, Peter & Balzarini, J & Egberink, H.F.. (2007). Antiviral activity of carbohydrate-binding agents against Nidovirales in cell culture. Antiviral research. 76. 21-9. 10.1016/j.antiviral.2007.04.003.

9 Yang Y, Islam MS, Wang J, Li Y, Chen X. Traditional Chinese Medicine in the Treatment of Patients Infected with 2019-New Coronavirus (SARS-CoV-2): A Review and Perspective. *Int J Biol Sci* 2020; 16(10):1708-1717. doi:10.7150/ijbs.45538. Available from http://www.ijbs.com/v16p1708.htm

10 Choi, Jang-Gi & Lee, Heeeun & Hwang, Youn-Hwan & Lee, Jong-Soo & Cho, Won-Kyung & Ma, Jin. (2017). Eupatorium fortunei and Its Components Increase Antiviral Immune Responses against RNA Viruses. Frontiers in Pharmacology. 8. 511. 10.3389/fphar.2017.00511.

11 Lara HH, Ayala-Nuñez NV, Ixtepan-Turrent L, Rodriguez-Padilla C. Mode of antiviral action of silver nanoparticles against HIV-1. *J Nanobiotechnology*. 2010;8:1. Published 2010 Jan 20. doi:10.1186/1477-3155-8-1

12 S. Ayehunie, A. Belay, T. W. Baba, and R. M. Ruprecht, "Inhibition of HIV-1 replication by an aqueous extract of *Spirulina platensis (Arthrospira platensis),*" *Journal of Acquired Immune Deficiency Syndromes and Human Retrovirology*, vol. 18, no. 1, pp. 7–12, 1998.

13 Lee-Huang S, Huang PL, Zhang D, et al. Discovery of small-molecule HIV-1 fusion and integrase inhibitors oleuropein and hydroxytyrosol: Part I. fusion [corrected] inhibition [published correction appears in Biochem Biophys Res Commun. 2007 May 18;356(4):1068]. *Biochem Biophys Res Commun*. 2007;354(4):872–878. doi:10.1016/j.bbrc.2007.01.071

14 Salehi B, Kumar NVA, Şener B, et al. Medicinal Plants Used in the Treatment of Human Immunodeficiency Virus. *Int J Mol Sci*. 2018;19(5):1459. Published 2018 May 14. doi:10.3390/ijms19051459

15 Jayakumar T, Hsieh CY, Lee JJ, Sheu JR. Experimental and Clinical Pharmacology of Andrographis paniculata and Its Major Bioactive Phytoconstituent Andrographolide. *Evid Based Complement Alternat Med*. 2013;2013:846740. doi:10.1155/2013/846740

16 Fink, R. C., Roschek, B., & Alberte, R. S. (2009). HIV Type-1 Entry Inhibitors with a New Mode of Action. Antiviral Chemistry and Chemotherapy, 243–255. https://doi.org/10.1177/095632020901900604

17 Lindequist U, Niedermeyer TH, Jülich WD. The pharmacological potential of mushrooms. *Evid Based Complement Alternat Med*. 2005;2(3):285–299. doi:10.1093/ecam/neh107

18 Chen CN, Lin CP, Huang KK, et al. Inhibition of SARS-CoV 3C-like Protease Activity by Theaflavin-3,3'-digallate (TF3). *Evid Based Complement Alternat Med*. 2005;2(2):209–215. doi:10.1093/ecam/neh081

Studies

Compendium of Clinical Studies Demonstrating Efficacy of Natural Compounds Against Coronaviruses

by Collin Gow, C.N.C. (3/18/2020)

"Griffithsin, a Highly Potent Broad-Spectrum Antiviral Lectin from Red Algae: From Discovery to Clinical Application"

"**GRFT is a red algae-derived lectin** of 121 amino acids (Figure 1). It exhibits potent (EC50 in the picomolar range) and broad-spectrum antiviral activity and negligible in vitro and in vivo host toxicity [9]. Its antiviral activity relates to a unique structural feature that forms a homodimeric complex with three carbohydrate-binding domains on each monomer (Figure 2). These three carbohydrate-binding domains **target high-mannose arrays present on many pathogenic enveloped viruses including** HIV; severe, acute, or **Middle East respiratory syndrome coronaviruses (SARS-CoV or MERS-CoV)** [10,11]; hepatitis C virus (HCV) [12,13]; herpes simplex virus 2 (HSV-2) [14,15]; Japanese encephalitis virus (JEV) [16,17]; and porcine epidemic diarrhea virus (PEDV) [18]. As a result of its broad antiviral spectrum, it shows great promise as a general microbicidal agent that can prevent viral transmission and as a therapeutic against enveloped virus-mediated diseases."

Lee, C. Griffithsin, a Highly Potent Broad-Spectrum Antiviral Lectin from Red Algae: From Discovery to Clinical Application. *Mar. Drugs* **2019**, *17*, 567.

"Antiviral Natural Products and Herbal Medicines"

"There are no specific treatments for CoV infection and preventive vaccines are still being explored. Thus, the situation reflects the need to develop effective antivirals for prophylaxis and treatment of CoV infection. We have previously reported that saikosaponins (A, B2, C, and D), which are **naturally** occurring triterpene glycosides isolated from medicinal plants such as *Bupleurum* spp. (柴胡 Chái Hú), *Heteromorpha* spp., and *Scrophularia scorodonia* (玄參 Xuán Shēn), exert antiviral activity against HCoV-22E9.[14] Upon co-challenge with the virus, **these natural compounds effectively prevent the early stage of HCoV-22E9 infection, including viral attachment and penetration.** Extracts from *Lycoris radiata* (石蒜 Shí Suàn), *Artemisia annua* (黃花蒿 Huáng Huā Hāo), *Pyrrosia lingua* (石葦 Shí Wěi), and *Lindera aggregata* (烏藥 Wū Yào) have also been documented to display **anti–SARS-CoV effect** from a screening analysis using hundreds of Chinese medicinal herbs.[15] **Natural inhibitors against the SARS-CoV enzymes, such as the nsP13 helicase and 3CL protease, have been identified as well and include myricetin, scutellarein, and phenolic compounds from** *Isatis indigotica* (板藍根 Bǎn Lán Gēn) and *Torreya nucifera* (榧 Fěi).[16,17,18] Other anti-CoV natural medicines include the water extract from *Houttuynia cordata* (魚腥草 Yú Xīng Cǎo), **which has been observed to exhibit several antiviral mechanisms against SARS-CoV, such as inhibiting the viral 3CL protease and blocking the viral RNA-dependent RNA polymerase activity.[19]"**

Lin, Liang-Tzung et al. "Antiviral natural products and herbal medicines." *Journal of traditional and complementary medicine* vol. 4,1 (2014): 24-35. doi:10.4103/2225-4110.124335

"Glycyrrhizin, an active component of liquorice roots, and replication of SARS-associated coronavirus."

"We assessed the antiviral potential of ribavirin, 6-azauridine, pyrazofurin, mycophenolic acid, and glycyrrhizin against two clinical isolates of coronavirus (FFM-1 and FFM-2) from patients with SARS admitted to the clinical centre of Frankfurt University, Germany. **Of all the compounds, glycyrrhizin [licorice] was the most active in inhibiting replication of the SARS-associated virus. Our findings suggest that glycyrrhizin should be assessed for treatment of SARS."**

Cinatl, J et al. "Glycyrrhizin, an active component of liquorice roots, and replication of SARS-associated coronavirus." *Lancet (London, England)* vol. 361,9374 (2003): 2045-6. doi:10.1016/s0140-6736(03)13615-x

"In vitro susceptibility of 10 clinical isolates of SARS coronavirus to selected antiviral compounds."

"**Commercial antiviral agents and pure chemical compounds extracted from traditional Chinese medicinal herbs were screened against 10 clinical isolates of SARS coronavirus by neutralisation tests with confirmation by plaque reduction assays.** Interferon-beta-1a, leukocytic interferon-alpha, ribavirin, lopinavir, rimantadine, **baicalin [Chinese skullcap] and glycyrrhizin [licorice] showed** antiviral activity."

Chen, F et al. "In vitro susceptibility of 10 clinical isolates of SARS coronavirus to selected antiviral compounds." *Journal of clinical virology : the official publication of the Pan American Society for Clinical Virology* vol. 31,1 (2004): 69-75. doi:10.1016/j.jcv.2004.03.003

"Small molecules targeting severe acute respiratory syndrome human coronavirus"

"**Compounds 5 (Aescin, a drug widely used in Europe) and 13** (Reserpine, a Food and Drug Administration-approved drug) **were further tested** with IFA, ELISA, Western blot analysis, and flow cytometry to confirm their anti-SARS activities. The EC50 values for Reserpine (compound **13**) and Aescin (compound **5**) were 3.4 μM and 6.0 μM, respectively, and the corresponding CC50 values were 25 μM (SI = 7.3) and 15 μM (SI = 2.5).

Aescin, the major active principle from the horse chestnut tree, has previously been used to treat patients with chronic venous insufficiency (30, 31), hemorrhoids (32), postoperative edema (30, 32), and inflammatory action (30, 33). Reserpine, a naturally occurring alkaloid produced by several members of the genus Rauwolfia, has been used primarily as a peripheral antihypertensive and as a central depressant and sedative (34). It has also found use as a radio-protective agent and experimentally as a contraceptive (35).

Because Glycyrrhizin, Aescin [horse chestnut] and Reserpine **have been used clinically, their related natural products may be also active against SARS-CoV.** We used the International Species Information System (ISIS) database to search for commercially available compounds whose structures have 80% similarities with these three drugs. We found 15 compounds related to Glycyrrhizin and Aescin and six compounds related to Reserpine. Through a cell-based assay, **we found that 10 of the 21 compounds showed activities against SARS-CoV. Among them, four compounds (6, 16, 17, and 18) are derivatives of Glycyrrhizin and Aescin, and all six derivatives of Reserpine (19–24) showed activities toward SARS-CoV at <100 μM.**

Some other well known traditional Chinese herbs were also tested in the cell-based assay and most of them were found inactive **against SARS-CoV** at the concentration of 10 μM. However, **we found that extracts of eucalyptus and *Lonicera japonica* did show such activities at the concentration of 100 μM; and Ginsenoside-Rb1 (17), one of the pharmacologically active components of Panax ginseng** (42, 43)

Finally, previous reports in the literature have predicted that several compounds may show antiviral activities against SARS, such as AG7088 (21), Pentoxifylline (45), **Melatonin (46), and Vitamin C (47). However, our cell-based assay showed that these compounds had no effects at the concentration of 10 μM.** Some other anti-RNA virus drugs, such as AZT, Didanosine, Nevirapine, Ritonavir, Lopinavir, Saquinavir, and Ribavirin, also showed no activities at the same concentration."

Wu, Chung-Yi et al. "Small molecules targeting severe acute respiratory syndrome human coronavirus." *Proceedings of the National Academy of Sciences of the United States of America* vol. 101,27 (2004): 10012-7. doi:10.1073/pnas.0403596101

"Identification of natural compounds with antiviral activities against SARS-associated coronavirus"

"After primary screening, active compounds were cherry picked and a second round of test was performed for their antiviral effects. The pictures were taken to record cell morphology change caused by CPE and the inhibition effects of the compounds before MTS assay. As shown in Fig. 1, **four of the extracts, Lycoris radiata, Artemisia annua, Pyrrosia lingua, and Lindera aggregata exhibited significant inhibition effects on virus-induced CPE when SARS-CoV strain BJ001 was used in screening.**
Out of the four, Lycoris radiata was most potent.
One of the active samples which showed better inhibition effect in anti-SARS-CoV screening, L. radiata extract, was chosen for further identification of the active component in it. We first isolated the total alkaloid from L. radiata according to previous reports (Hong and Ma, 1964). We then examined its antiviral activity. This was based on previous findings that the majority of bioactive components of L. radiata were from its alkaloid fraction (Takagi et al., 1968; Miyasaka and Hiramatsu, 1980; Cortese et al., 1983). **From CPE/MTS assays, the isolated alkaloid showed potent inhibitory activity against SARS-CoV infection"**

Li, Shi-You et al. "Identification of natural compounds with antiviral activities against SARS-associated coronavirus." *Antiviral research* vol. 67,1 (2005): 18-23. doi:10.1016/j.antiviral.2005.02.007

"Herbal plants and plant preparations as remedial approach for viral diseases"

"Dioscorea Extracts. Patent No. US 20090041803; Filed September 02, 2008 [106]
This extract is an immunogenic composition that contains an antigen agent and an adjuvant agent, wherein the adjuvant agent contains an extract that is prepared from a tuber of a Dioscorea plant. This extract is prepared from the tuber of any of these **Dioscorea species namely D. batatas, D. ecne, D. alata L., D. pseudojaponica, or D. alata L. var. purpurea.** The antigen agent can be a polypeptide, such as a viral protein or a tumor antigen protein or a nucleic acid encoding the polypeptide. The invention is useful in but not limited to treating viral diseases such as infection by an adenovirus, a herpesvirus (e.g., HSV-I, HSV-II, CMV, or VZV), a poxvirus (e.g., an orthopoxvirus such as variola or vaccinia, or molluscum contagiosum), a picornavirus (e.g., rhinovirus or enterovirus), an orthomyxovirus (e.g., influenzavirus), a paramyxovirus [e.g., parainfluenzavirus, mumps virus, measles virus, and respiratory syncytial virus (RSV)], **a coronavirus (e.g., SARS)**, a papovavirus (e.g., papillomaviruses, such as those that cause genital warts, common warts, or plantar warts), a hepadnavirus (e.g., hepatitis B virus), a flavivirus (e.g., hepatitis C virus or Dengue virus), or a retrovirus (e.g., a lentivirus such as HIV). This herbal preparation also can be used as a dietary supplement, health food, or health drink for prevention of immune system impairment. It also finds use in treating a range of bacterial, fungal and neoplastic diseases."

Ganjhu, Rajesh Kumar et al. "Herbal plants and plant preparations as remedial approach for viral diseases." *Virusdisease* vol. 26,4 (2015): 225-36. doi:10.1007/s13337-015-0276-6

"Potential antivirals and antiviral strategies against SARS coronavirus infections."

"**Various other compounds**, often with an ill-defined mode of action but selectivity indexes up to 100, **have been reported to exhibit** *in vitro* **activity against SARS-CoV:** valinomycin, glycopeptide antibiotics, plant lectins, **hesperetin**, glycyrrhizin, aurintricarboxylic acid, chloroquine, niclosamide, nelfinavir and calpain inhibitors.
Inhibitory effects on SARS-CoV replication, with selectivity indexes of up to 100, and EC50 values as low as 1 µg/ml, **have been observed for a variety of compounds including** the vancomycin, eremomycin and teicoplanin aglycon derivatives [70], and the **mannose-specific plant lectins derived from** *G. nivalis*, *Hippeastrum hybrid*[71] **and** *Allium porrum* (leek) [72]. The mode of action of these compounds has not been assessed, but it is tempting to speculate that they interfere with the binding of the S glycoprotein to the host cells.
Isatis indigotica **root and phenolic Chinese herbs were frequently used for the prevention of SARS during the SARS outbreaks in China, Hong Kong and Taiwan.** *I. indigotica* root (*Radix isatidis*) is native to China. **From the** *I. indigotica* **root extracts several compounds, that is, indigo, sinigrin, aloe-emodin and hesperetin, were isolated that inhibited the cell-free and cell-based cleavage activity of the SARS Mpro (3CLpro)** at IC50 values ranging from 10 to 1000 µM [73]. The inhibitory effects on SARS-CoV replication in cell culture (i.e., Vero cells) were not determined in this study. The cytotoxicity was determined, however, and, based on the ratio of the CC50 to the IC50 (cell-based cleavage), **hesperetin appeared to be the most selective** (selectivity index: ~300) [73]."

De Clercq, Erik. "Potential antivirals and antiviral strategies against SARS coronavirus infections." *Expert review of anti-infective therapy* vol. 4,2 (2006): 291-302. doi:10.1586/14787210.4.2.291

"Antiviral activity of carbohydrate-binding agents against Nidovirales in cell culture"

"Coronaviruses are important human and animal pathogens, the relevance of which increased due **to the emergence of new human coronaviruses like SARS-CoV, HKU1 and NL63. Together with toroviruses, arteriviruses, and roniviruses the coronaviruses belong to the order** *Nidovirales*. **So far antivirals are hardly available to combat infections with viruses of this order.** Therefore, various antiviral strategies to counter nidoviral infections are under evaluation. Lectins, which bind to N-linked oligosaccharide elements of enveloped viruses, can be considered as a conceptionally new class of virus inhibitors. These agents were recently evaluated for their antiviral activity towards a variety of enveloped viruses and were shown in most cases to inhibit virus infection at low concentrations. However, limited knowledge is available for their efficacy towards nidoviruses. **In this article the application of the plant lectins *Hippeastrum* hybrid agglutinin (HHA), *Galanthus nivalis* agglutinin (GNA), *Cymbidium* sp. agglutinin (CA) and *Urtica dioica* agglutinin (UDA) as well as non-plant derived pradimicin-A (PRM-A) and cyanovirin-N (CV-N) as potential antiviral agents was evaluated.** Three antiviral tests were compared based on different evaluation principles: cell viability (MTT-based colorimetric assay), number of infected cells (immunoperoxidase assay) and amount of viral protein expression (luciferase-based assay). **The presence of carbohydrate-binding agents strongly inhibited coronaviruses (transmissible gastroenteritis virus, infectious bronchitis virus, feline coronaviruses serotypes I and II, mouse hepatitis virus), arteriviruses (equine arteritis virus and porcine respiratory and reproductive syndrome virus) and torovirus (equine Berne virus).** Remarkably, serotype II feline coronaviruses and arteriviruses were not inhibited by PRM-A, in contrast to the other viruses tested.

"We were able to show for UDA [*Urtica dioica* agglutinin] [stinging nettle rhizome] also a high antiviral efficacy against all evaluated *Nidovirales* except PRRSV."

van der Meer, F J U M et al. "Antiviral activity of carbohydrate-binding agents against Nidovirales in cell culture." *Antiviral research* vol. 76,1 (2007): 21-9. doi:10.1016/j.antiviral.2007.04.003

"An unusual lectin from stinging nettle (Urtica dioica) rhizomes"

"UDA induced considerable amounts of antiviral activity in the cell cultures. Moreover, the antiviral activity produced after stimulating lymphocytes with UDA was characterized by using specific antisera as being due solely to HuIFN-y (formerly called immune interferon)."

Peumans, Willy J. et al. "An unusual lectin from stinging nettle (Urtica dioica) rhizomes." *FEBS Letters* 177 (1984): n. pag.

"Effective inhibition of MERS-CoV infection by resveratrol"

"Resveratrol significantly inhibited MERS-CoV infection and prolonged cellular survival after virus infection. We also found that the expression of nucleocapsid (N) protein essential for MERS-CoV replication was decreased after resveratrol treatment. Furthermore, resveratrol down-regulated the apoptosis induced by MERS-CoV in vitro. By consecutive administration of resveratrol, we were able to reduce the concentration of resveratrol while achieving inhibitory effectiveness against MERS-CoV."

"In this study, we first demonstrated that resveratrol is a potent anti-MERS agent in vitro. We perceive that resveratrol can be a potential antiviral agent against MERS-CoV infection in the

near future."

Lin, Shih-Chao et al. "Effective inhibition of MERS-CoV infection by resveratrol." *BMC infectious diseases* vol. 17,1 144. 13 Feb. 2017, doi:10.1186/s12879-017-2253-8

"In vitro antiviral activity of fifteen plant extracts against avian infectious bronchitis virus"

"IB is a highly contagious respiratory and occasionally urogenital disease in chickens [1]. **IBV affects the upper respiratory tract** and reduces egg production [2]. **It is a coronavirus that belongs to the *Coronaviridae* family. IBV is an enveloped virus with a single-stranded positive-sense linear RNA molecule (approximately 27.6 kb in size) [3].**

IB has a wide geographical distribution and is diagnosed worldwide [1]. IB outbreaks continuously and results in economic losses in the poultry industry. **So far vaccination using inactivated or live vaccines [4] is regarded as the main method of prevention, but it is not having the desired effect [5,6,7]. The high level of mutations of IBV [8] leads to the emergence of new serotypes and genotypes, and limits the efficacy of routine prevention.**

Antiviral effect against IBV

According to the results of the antiviral effect assay, eight extracts were selected for determination of the virucidal effect. **The selected extracts of *S. montana, O. vulgare, M. piperita, M. officinalis, T. vulgaris, H. officinalis, S. officinalis* and *D. canadense* showed anti-IBV activity in two of the four methods. All eight extracts showed an antiviral effect prior to infection (method 1). Furthermore, seven of these showed antiviral activity during infection (method 2), while only the extract of *S. montana* [*Satureja montana*] [winter savory] showed anti-IBV activity after infection (method 4). *P. frutescens, N. cataria, E. purpurea, Ch. nobile* and *A. foeniculum* showed an antiviral effect only in the first method, while *G. macrorrhizum* and *A. archangelica* did not show an antiviral effect in any method (Table 1).**

The above-mentioned eight plant extracts demonstrating anti-IBV activity were selected for further investigation. The 50% effective concentration (EC50) was determined in cells grown for 4 days (prior to infection). The EC50 values of extracts of *S. montana, O. vulgare* [oregano], *M. piperita* [peppermint], *M. officinalis* [lemon balm], *T. vulgaris* [thyme], *H. officinalis, S. officinalis* and *D. canadense* were between 0.003 and 0.076 μg, however **S. officinalis** [*Salvia officinalis*] **appeared effective at the lowest concentration (0.003 μg)** (Table 2). SI of *M. piperita, O. vulgare,* and *T. vulgaris* extracts were 67.5, 65.0 and 63.1 respectively."

Lelešius, Raimundas & Karpovaitė, Agneta & Mickienė, Rūta & Drevinskas, Tomas & Tiso, Nicola & Ragazinskiene, Ona & Kubilienė, Loreta & Maruska, Audrius & Salomskas, Algirdas. (2019). In vitro antiviral activity of fifteen plant extracts against avian infectious bronchitis virus. BMC Veterinary Research. 15. 10.1186/s12917-019-1925-6.

"Traditional Chinese Medicine in the Treatment of Patients Infected with 2019-New Coronavirus (SARS-CoV-2): A Review and Perspective"

"There are quite compelling evidences support the notion that TCM has beneficial effect in the treatment or prevention of SARS. For example, the rate of fatality in Hong Kong and Singapore was approximately 18%, while the rate for Beijing was initially more than 52% until the 5th of May and decreased gradually to 4%-1% after the 20th of May in 2003. The dramatic reduced fatality from late May in Beijing was believed to be associated with the use of TCM as a supplement to the conventional therapy [44]. Lau and colleagues reported that, during SARS outbreak, 1063 volunteers including 926 hospital workers and 37 laboratory technicians working in high-risk virus laboratories used a TCM herbal extract, namely *Sang Ju Yin* plus *Yu Ping Feng San*. Compared with the 0.4% of infection in the control group, none of TCM users infected. Furthermore, there was some evidence that *Sang Ju Yin* plus *Yu Ping Feng San* could modulate T cells in a manner to enhance host defense capacity [45, 46]. In a controlled clinical study, the supplementary treatment with TCM resulted in marked improvement of symptoms and shortened the disease course [47]. The clinical beneficial effect of TCM appears to be supported by laboratory studies."

C   🔒 ijbs.com/v16p1708.htm   ☆ ⬡

TCM Compound (s)	Mode of action	Reference
Plant-derived phenolic compounds and Root extract of *Isatis indigotica*	Inhibit the cleavage activity of SARS-3CLpro enzyme	[57]
Water extract of *Houttuynia cordata*	Inhibit the viral SARS-3CLpro activity Block viral RNA-dependent RNA polymerase activity (RdRp) Immunomodulation	[54, 55]
Scutellarein and myricetin	Inhibit nsP13 by affecting the ATPase activity	[61]
Glycyrrhizin from *Glycyrrhizae radix*	Inhibit viral adsorption and penetration	[48, 73]
Herbacetin, quercetin, isobavaschalcone, 3-β-D-glucoside and helichrysetin	Inhibit cleavage activity of MERS-3CLpro enzyme	[60]
Tetrandrine, fangchinoline, and cepharanthine	Inhibit the expression of HCoV-OC43 spike and nucleocapsid protein. Immunomodulation	[106, 119]
Chinese Rhubarb extracts	Inhibit SARS-3CLpro activity	[53]
Flavonoids (For example: extracted from litchi seeds, herbacetin, rhoifolin, pectolinarin, quercetin, epigallocatechin gallate, and gallocatechin gallate)	Inhibit SARS-3CLpro activity	[56, 58, 59]
Quercetin and TSL-1 from *Toona sinensis* Roem	Inhibit the cellular entry of SARS-CoV	[76]
Emodin derived from genus *Rheum* and *Polygonum*	Inhibit interaction of SARS-CoV Spike protein and ACE2 Inhibit the 3a ion channel of coronavirus SARS-CoV and HCoV-OC43	[67, 72]
Kaempferol derivatives	Inhibit 3a ion channel of coronavirus	[73]
Baicalin from *Scutellaria baicalensis*	Inhibit Angiotensin-converting enzyme (ACE)	[44, 68]
Saikosaponins	Prevent the early stage of HCoV-22E9 infection, including viral attachment and penetration	[74]
Tetra-O-galloyl-β-D-glucose and luteolin, from *Galla chinensis* and *Veronicalina niifolia* respectively	Avidly binds with surface spike protein of SARS-CoV	[71]

"The helicase protein is also considered as a potential target for the development of anti-HCoV (human coronavirus) agents. Yu *et al.* reported **scutellarein and myricetin potently inhibited the nsP13 (SARS-CoV helicase protein)** *in vitro* **by affecting the ATPase activity** [61]. The RNA- dependent RNA polymerase (RdRp), a key enzyme responsible for both positive and negative-strand RNA synthesis, also represents another potential druggable target. It was shown that the **extracts of *Kang***

100

Du Bu Fei Tang (IC50:471.3 µg/mL), *Sinomenium acutum* (IC50:198.6 µg/mL), *Coriolus versicolor* [turkey tail mushroom] (IC50:108.4 µg/mL) and *Ganoderma lucidum* [reishi] (IC50:41.9 µg/mL) inhibited SARS-CoV RdRp in a dose- dependent manner [54]. Wu *et al.* performed large- scale screening of existing drugs, natural products, and synthetic compounds (>10000 compounds) to identify effective anti-SARS-CoV agents through a cell-based assay with SARS virus and Vero E6 cells [62]. They found that ginsenoside-Rb1 isolated from *Panax ginseng*, aescin isolated from the horse chestnut tree, reserpine contained in the genus *Rauwolfia* and extracts of *eucalyptus* and *Lonicera japonica* inhibited SARS-CoV replication at non-toxic concentrations [62].

Same as SARS-CoV and HCoV-NL63, SARS-CoV-2 uses host receptor ACE2 for the cellular entrance [63-66]. Therefore, TCM with the capacity to target ACE2 holds the promise to prevent the infection of SARS-CoV-2. Emodin from genus *Rheum* and *Polygonum* [67], baicalin from in *Scutellaria baicalensis* [44, 68], **nicotianamine from foodstuff (especially "soybean ACE2 inhibitor (ACE2iSB)")** [69], scutellarin [70], tetra-*O*-galloyl-β-D-glucose (TGG) from *Galla chinensis* and luteolin from *Veronicalina riifolia* [71] markedly inhibited the interaction of SARS-CoV S-protein and ACE2. However, the anti-SARS-CoV activity of these compounds remain to be evaluated. In addition, inhibition of the 3a ion channel by emodin [72] or kaempferol derivatives-juglanin [73] could potentially prevent the viral release from the infected cells. **Saikosaponins [74], glycyrrhizin [48, 75], quercetin and TSL-1 extracted from *Toona sinensis* Roem [76] purportedly had potent anti-SARS-CoV effects by inhibition of viral cellular entry, adsorption, and penetration.**

Overwhelming inflammatory responses are attributable to the deaths of patients with infection of SARS-CoV, or MERS-CoV, or COVID-19. Thus, anti-inflammatory agents presumably could reduce the severity and mortality rate [77]. *Shuang Huang Lian,* **a TCM herbal product prepared from *Lonicerae japonicae* Flos, *Scutellariae radix* and *Fructus Forsythiae,* purportedly had the activity to inhibit SARS-CoV-2 [78]. Interestingly, We have shown that this herbal preparation potently inhibited staphylococcal toxic shock syndrome toxin 1 (TSST-1)-induced production of cytokines (IL-1β, IL-6, TNF-α, IFN-γ) and chemokines (MIP-1α, MIP-1β and MCP-1) by peripheral blood mononuclear cell (PBMC) [79]. In line with our results, this herbal product was shown to markedly reduced the transcriptional and translational levels of inflammatory cytokines TNF-α, IL-1β, and IL-6 in lipopolysaccharide-stimulated murine alveolar macrophages [80].** Indirubin is an active ingredient of a TCM preparation *Dang Gui Long Hui Pill,* had strong antiviral and immunomodulatory effects, as shown by a study based on the observation of influenza H5N1 virus-infected human macrophages and type-I alveolar epithelial cells [81]. *Lian Hua Qing Wen* **Capsule was reported to have *in vitro* activity in inhibition of propagation of various influenza viruses. This TCM herbal product not only blocked the early stages of influenza virus infection but also inhibited virus-induced gene expression of IL-6, IL-8, TNF-a, IP-10, and MCP-1 [82]. Additionally, a study by Dong *et al.* reported that the levels of IL-8, TNF-α, IL-17, and IL-23 in the sputum and of IL-8 and IL-17 in the blood were markedly decreased after *Lian Hua Qing Wen Capsule* treatment in patients with acute exacerbation of chronic obstructive pulmonary disease [83].** A self-control study by Poon *et al.* showed that the administration of the TCM herbal formulas (*Sang Ju Yin* and *Yu Ping Feng San*) may have beneficial immunomodulatory effects for the prevention of viral infections including SARS-CoV [46].

Moreover, a number of anti-coronaviral agents have been identified from TCM herbs, although the mechanisms of action have not yet been elucidated. For example, extracts from *Lycoris radiata, Artemisia annua, Pyrrosia lingua*, and *Lindera aggregate* possessed the anti-SARS-CoV activity [84], **3β-Friedelanol isolated from *Euphorbia neriifolia* [85], Blancoxanthone isolated from** the roots of *Calophyllum blancoi* [86] exhibited anti-HCoV-229E activity."

Yang, Yang et al. "Traditional Chinese Medicine in the Treatment of Patients Infected with 2019-New Coronavirus (SARS-CoV-2): A Review and Perspective." *International journal of biological sciences* vol. 16,10 1708-1717. 15 Mar. 2020, doi:10.7150/ijbs.45538

"Echinacea—A Source of Potent Antivirals for Respiratory Virus Infections"

Table 1

Respiratory viruses and their potential targets.

Virus	Relevant properties	Potential targets	Susceptible to Echinacea(±)[1]
Influenza viruses A & B (FluV A/B) (Orthomyxoviridae)	Segmented ssRNA genome + membrane	Hemagglutinin, neuraminidase (others ?)	+
Respiratory syncytial virus (RSV) (Paramyxoviridae)	ssRNA + membrane	Membrane components	+
Parainfluenza viruses (PI 1-4), (Paramyxoviridae)	ssRNA + membrane	Membrane components	?
Metapneumoviruses (hMPV) (Paramyxoviridae)	ssRNA + membrane	Membrane components	?
Coronaviruses (HCoV, SARS CoV) (Coronaviridae)	ssRNA + membrane	Membrane components	+
Rhinoviruses, coxsackieviruses, (Picornaviridae)	ssRNA, no membrane	Capsid proteins, replication	+
Adenoviruses (Adenoviridae)	dsDNA, no membrane	Capsid proteins, replication	-
Herpes viruses HSV-1/2 (Herpesviridae)	dsDNA + membrane	Membrane components virus replication	+
Bocavirus (HBoV) (Parvoviridae)	ssDNA, no membrane	Capsid proteins	?

[1] details and references in text (Section 3)

Hudson, James, and Selvarani Vimalanathan. "Echinacea—A Source of Potent Antivirals for Respiratory Virus Infections." *Pharmaceuticals* vol. 4,7 1019–1031. 13 Jul. 2011, doi:10.3390/ph4071019

"High-Throughput Screening and Identification of Potent Broad-Spectrum Inhibitors of Coronaviruses"

"Furthermore, we identified seven compounds (**lycorine**, emetine, monensin sodium, mycophenolate mofetil, mycophenolic acid, phenazopyridine, and pyrvinium pamoate) as **broad-spectrum inhibitors according to their strong inhibition of replication by four CoVs *in vitro* at low-micromolar** concentrations. Additionally, we found that emetine blocked MERS-CoV entry according to pseudovirus entry assays and that lycorine protected BALB/c mice against HCoV-OC43-induced lethality by decreasing viral load in the central nervous system. **This represents the first demonstration of *in vivo* real-time bioluminescence imaging to monitor the effect of lycorine on the spread and distribution of HCoV-OC43 in a mouse model. These results offer critical information supporting the development of an effective therapeutic strategy against CoV infection.**"

Shen, Liang et al. "High-Throughput Screening and Identification of Potent Broad-Spectrum Inhibitors of Coronaviruses." *Journal of virology* vol. 93,12 e00023-19. 29 May. 2019, doi:10.1128/JVI.00023-19

"*Eupatorium fortunei* and Its Components Increase Antiviral Immune Responses against RNA Viruses"

"Also, according to recent research results, **quercetin has been shown to protect against** the entry of influenza A virus (Wu et al., 2015) and interaction between human respiratory syncytial virus M2-1 protein (Teixeira et al., 2017), have anti-HSV-1 and anti-HSV-2 properties (Lee et al., 2017), **and inhibit coronavirus** and dengue virus infection (Chiow et al., 2016)."

Choi, Jang-Gi et al. "*Eupatorium fortunei* and Its Components Increase Antiviral Immune Responses against RNA Viruses." *Frontiers in pharmacology* vol. 8 511. 3 Aug. 2017, doi:10.3389/fphar.2017.00511

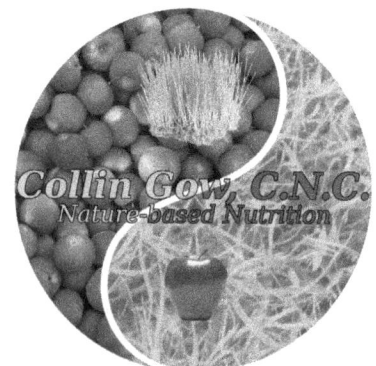

Probiotics and the Neurotransmitters, Hormones, Enzymes, Antioxidants, and Vitamins They Produce

by Collin Gow, C.N.C.

GABA producers: paracasei, delbrukii, bulgaricus, lactis, brevis, longum

Lowers cortisol: infantis

Tryptophan producers: infantis, Candida, Streptococcus, Escherichia, Enterococcus

Superoxide dismutase producer: thermophilus

Histamine producers: proteus, E. coli, Staphylococci

Eliminate nitrates: longum

Urinary tract/vagina health: reuteri, rhamnosus, crispatus

Increase lymphocytes: Bifidobacteria

Iron robbing: Actinomyces, Mycobacterium, E. coli, Corynebacterium

Increase dopamine: Bacillus

Alcohol producer: Candida

Increase nitric oxide: plantarum, subtilis

Proteolytic: faecalis TH10

Sulphite producing: Proteobacteria, Thiobacilli, Chromatiacea, Desufotomaculum

Hemolytic: Streptococcus parasanguinis, Gamella hemolysans

ACE inhibiting: helveticus, plantarum

Lower triglycerides: plantarum

Fibrinolytic: Treponema, subtilis

Lowers fibrinogen: coagulans

C. Diff fighter: boulardii, subtilis

MRSA fighter: boulardii, subtilis

Candida fighter: coagulans, subtilis

Glutathione producer: fermentum ME-3

Vitamin K2 producer: subtilis

Available for download @ collingowcnc.wixsite.com/collingowcnc/articlesandprotocols

References:

1. http://www.gastrojournal.org/article/S0016-5085(11)00607-X/fulltext
2. http://www.ncbi.nlm.nih.gov/pmc/articles/PMC3182331/

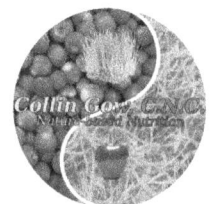

3. http://onlinelibrary.wiley.com/doi/10.1111/j.1365-2036.2012.05104.x/full#apt5104-sec-0015

4. Videlock, E. J. and Cremonini, F. (2012), Meta-analysis: probiotics in antibiotic-associated diarrhoea. Alimentary Pharmacology & Therapeutics, 35: 1355–1369. doi: 10.1111/j.1365-2036.2012.05104.x

5. Hawrelak, JA. (ed). Probiotic Advisor. Illuminate Natural Medicine, 2015 https://www.probioticadvisor.com/advisor/. Accessed 30 September 2015.

6. http://www.ncbi.nlm.nih.gov/pubmed/21114493

7. http://www.ncbi.nlm.nih.gov/pubmed/11799281

8. http://drprobiotikum.hu/docs/synbiotics-in-managment-of-infantile%20colic.pdf

9. http://www.ncbi.nlm.nih.gov/pubmed/20974015

10. http://www.ncbi.nlm.nih.gov/pmc/articles/PMC3446166/

11. http://www.tandfonline.com/doi/full/10.4161/gmic.28682

12. Elaine Patterson, John F. Cryan, Gerald F. Fitzgerald, R. Paul Ross, Timothy G. Dinan and Catherine Stanton (2014). Gut microbiota, the pharmabiotics they produce and host health. Proceedings of the Nutrition Society, 73, pp 477-489. doi:10.1017/S0029665114001426.

13. http://moldrecovery.blogspot.com/2011/02/health-benefits-of-lacto-fermented.html#.VqqZnfkrLak

14. https://www.psychologytoday.com/blog/evolutionary-psychiatry/201206/groovy-probiotics

15. Clark, L. C. and Hodgkin, J. (2014), Commensals in the C. elegans model. Cell Microbiol, 16: 27-38. doi:10.1111/cmi.12234

16. Schnorr, Stephanie L et al. "Gut microbiome of the Hadza hunter-gatherers." Nature communications vol. 5 3654. 15 Apr. 2014, doi:10.1038/ncomms4654

17. https://www.ncbi.nlm.nih.gov/pubmed/16232939

18. Hu, Yuanliang et al. "Purification and characterization of a novel, highly potent fibrinolytic enzyme from Bacillus subtilis DC27 screened from Douchi, a traditional Chinese fermented soybean food." Scientific reports vol. 9,1 9235. 25 Jun. 2019, doi:10.1038/s41598-019-45686-y

19. Abhari, Khadijeh et al. "The effects of orally administered Bacillus coagulans and inulin on prevention and progression of rheumatoid arthritis in rats." Food & nutrition research vol. 60 30876. 15 Jul. 2016, doi:10.3402/fnr.v60.30876

20. Tung, Jennifer M et al. "Prevention of Clostridium difficile infection with Saccharomyces boulardii: a systematic review." Canadian journal of gastroenterology = Journal canadien de gastroenterologie vol. 23,12 (2009): 817-21. doi:10.1155/2009/915847

21. Colenutt, C. and Cutting, S. M. (2014), Use of Bacillus subtilis PXN21 spores for suppression of Clostridium difficile infection symptoms in a murine model. FEMS Microbiol Lett, 358: 154-161. doi:10.1111/1574-6968.12468

22. Sizemore, Elizabeth Nicole et al. "Enteral vancomycin and probiotic use for methicillin-resistant Staphylococcus aureus antibiotic-associated diarrhoea." BMJ case reports vol. 2012 bcr2012006366. 27 Jul. 2012, doi:10.1136/bcr-2012-006366

23. Piewngam, Pipat et al. "Pathogen elimination by probiotic Bacillus via signalling interference." Nature vol. 562,7728 (2018): 532-537. doi:10.1038/s41586-018-0616-y

24. Mikelsaar, Marika, and Mihkel Zilmer. "Lactobacillus fermentum ME-3 - an antimicrobial and antioxidative probiotic." Microbial ecology in health and disease vol. 21,1 (2009): 1-27. doi:10.1080/08910600902815561

25. https://www.ncbi.nlm.nih.gov/pubmed/30882242

The Amazing Scientific Evidence on Butyrate for Gut Health and Beyond

Butyrate is an essential short chain fatty acid (SCFA) metabolite, aka "postbiotic", produced in the body by the fermentation of fiber by gut microbiota. It's the primary source of energy for colon cells[1,2], supports normal intestinal PH[1], assists in modulating innate immunity[3], upregulates the expression of and assembly of tight-junction proteins,[1,2,4,5,6,7,8] supports intestinal mucosa homeostasis,[2,3] and so much more. Fiber is very good for you, but some people have problems increasing fiber in their diets due to gas, bloating, pain, constipation and so on. Butyrate is a good solution to this problem as it gives you some of the benefits of fermentable fibers (prebiotics), without the side effects, as it contains no fiber. It may also give you some of the benefits of probiotics, without containing any bacteria. This makes butyrate an especially good, safe, and mild, but effective choice for those with leaky gut or other digestive issues. Butyrate has over 50,000 mentions in the medical literature, however, and a vast array of documented benefits for humans, from gut, to brain, to bones, to immune, to reducing inflammation and fat accumulation, to skin health, and beyond. This exposé presents only a small portion of the scientific evidence of its favorable effects on the body.

More on short chain fatty acids (SCFAs): as metabolic byproducts of fermentation, SCFAs can be called postbiotics. Nearly all the benefits for the host that are conferred by probiotics comes from the fact that they produce postbiotics. SCFAs are some of the most important postbiotics. Acetic acid, proprionic acid, and butyric acid are the most abundant SCFAs in the colon, making up 90-95%.[9] The amino acids valine, leucine, and isoleucine can be converted into the SCFAs isobutyrate, isovalerate, and 2-methylbutyrate, but make up a very small portion (5%) of total SCFA production.[9] Acetate is the most abundant SCFA in the colon and makes up over half of the total SCFAs in feces.[9] Short chain fatty acid ratios in the colon lumen are approximately 60% acetate, 25% proprionate, and 15% butyrate.[10] Others say 60:20:20.[11] Yet, butyrate appears to be the most important in the colon as it is the major energy source for colonocytes, while proprionate is mostly taken up by the liver and acetate enters circulation and is metabolized by various peripheral tissues.[12] 60-70% of the energy requirements of colon epithelial cells come from SCFAs and 5-15% of total caloric requirements of humans come from SCFAs.[13] Members of the *Lachnospiraceae* and *Ruminococcaceae* and some *Bacteroidetes* Families are the primary butyrate producers found in humans. The two most prevalent species of butyrate producing microbiota in humans are *Faecalibacterium prausnitzii* and *Eubacterium rectale/Roseburia* spp., both from *Clostridial* clusters.[14] Other microbiota such as *Clostridium butyricum*, are capable butyrate producers as well.

Butyrate is a salt or ester of butyric acid and is the form present in dietary supplements. Butyrate can be found in different forms such as calcium butyrate, magnesium butyrate, or sodium butyrate.

Scientific Evidence on Butyric Acid and Butyrate

Butyric acid:
- **Regulates transepithelial transport**[15]
- **Modulates motility**[15]
- May prevent and inhibit colon carcinoma[15]

- **Enhances absorptive** and antisecretive **capabilities of intestinal mucosa**[15]
- **Increases expression of mucin genes** and stimulates production of mucin[15]
- **Inhibits NF-κB and reduces expression of cytokine genes TNFα, IL1β, IL2, IL6, IL8, and IL12**[15]
- **Reduces reactive oxygen species**[15]
- **Increases amount of reduced glutathione**[15]

Butyrate:
- **Fuels intestinal epithelial cells**[9]
- Increases mucin production[9]
- **Improves tight-junction integrity**[9]
- **Reduces obesity and insulin resistance**[9]
- **Promotes a change from lipid synthesis to lipid oxidation**[9]
- **May activate AMP-k or MAPK**[9]
- **Induces production of gut hormones reducing food intake**[9]
- Protects against development of colorectal cancer[9]
- **Promotes colon motility**[9]
- **Reduces inflammation**[9]
- Increases visceral irrigation[9]
- Induces apoptosis[9]
- **Inhibits tumor cell progression**[9]
- **Inhibits histone deacetylation**[9]
- **Induces the differentiation of T-regulatory cells**[9]
- **Assists in controlling intestinal inflammation**[9]
- **May reduce the risk of inflammatory bowel disease**[9]
- **Gut barrier maintanence**[9]
- **Preferred energy source for colon epithelial cells**[1]
- Decreases the PH of the colon (a good thing) which **increases bile salt solubility, increases mineral absorption, decreases ammonia absorption, inhibits growth of pathogens**[1]
- Stimulates proliferation of colon epithelial cells[1]
- Reduces the proliferation and induces apoptosis of colorectal cancer cells[1]
- Affects gene expression of colon epithelial cells[1]
- **Plays a protective role against** colon cancer and **colitis**[1]
- **Improves gut barrier function** by stimulation of the formation of mucin, antimicrobial peptides, and tight-junction proteins[1]
- Interacts with the immune system[1]
- **Has anti-inflammatory effects**[1]
- **Stimulates the absorption of water and sodium**[1]
- **Reduces oxidative stress in the colon**[1]
- **Promotes satiety**[1]
- Reduces appetite[16]
- **Stimulates the metabolic activity of brown adipose tissue**[16]
- Enhances mitochondrial respiration of colonocytes[17]

- **Prevents colonocyte autophagy** (catabolic self-eating)[17]
- **Prevents adhesion of antigen-presenting cells**[18]
- Inhibit the proliferation and activation of T cells[18]
- **Improves neuroinflammation in aging mice** (attenuates pro-inflammatory cytokine expression in microglia)[19]
- Limits intestinal inflammation by **promoting the formation of regulatory T cells**[3]
- **Modulates the function of innate immune cells**[3]
- Inhibits histone deacetylases[3]
- Activates a receptor for niacin in the colon[3]
- Promotes expression of the pro-homeostatic cytokine IL-18[3]
- Increases colonic epithelial cell oxygen consumption (a good thing)[3]
- **Supports normal intestinal barrier function**[3]
- Plays a role in maintaining healthy colon barrier function[3]
- Promotes and maintains mucosal homeostasis[3]
- Regulates transepithelial fluid transport[2]
- Ameliorates mucosal inflammation and oxidative status[2]
- Reinforces epithelial defense barrier[2]
- **Modulates** visceral sensitivity and **intestinal motility**[2]
- Prevents and inhibits colorectal cancer[2]
- Potentially useful effects on hemoglobinopathies, genetic metabolic diseases, hypercholesterolemia, insulin resistance, and ischemic stroke[2]
- **Major energy source for colonocytes**[2]
- Stimulates sodium chloride absorption at the intestinal level[2]
- Increases WAF1 gene expression[2]
- Downregulates NRP-1[2]
- **Inhibits NF-κB in human colonic epithelial cells** which regulates genes involved in inflammatory responses such as IL-1b, TNF-α, IL-2, IL-6, IL-8, IL-12, iNOS, COX-2, ICAM-1, VCAM-1, TCR-α, and MHC class II molecules[2]
- **NF-κB is frequently disregulated in colon cancer, inflammatory bowel disease, ulcerative colitis, Chron's disease**[2]
- Decreases proinflammatory cytokine expression[2]
- Upregulates PPARγ and inhibits IFNγ signaling reducing inflammation[2]
- **Modulates oxidative stress in colonic mucosa**[2]
- Increases the expression of the MUC2 gene stimulating mucin production and enhancing protection against luminal agents[2]
- **Decreases intestinal cell permeability by assembling tight-junction** via AMPK[2]
- Regulates colonic mucosa homeostasis[2]
- **Modulates neuronal excitability**[2]
- Significantly increases the proportion of choline acetyltransferase and increases the cholinergic-mediated colonic circular muscle contractile response which may help with gastric motility[2]
- **Increases compliance, reduces pain, reduces urge, and reduces discomfort during rectal barostat procedure suggesting potential beneficial effect in IBS**[2]
- Reduced insulin resistance by 50% in mouse study[2]
- Postbiotic[2]

- Controls immune/inflammatory reactions in the skin applied topically and mediates ongoing contact hypersensitivity[20]
- Anti-inflammatory effect by activating G-protein-coupled receptors and inhibiting histone deacetylases[21]
- One of the major metabolites of gut microbiota[21]
- **Maintains homeostasis in the gut**[21]
- **Inhibits osteoclastogenesis which may reduce bone destruction** which is directly related to RA prognosis[21]
- **Antiinflammatory effect by downregulating IL-12 and upregulating IL-10**[21]
- **Ameliorates autoimmune** diseases such as experimental allergic encephalomyelitis, GvHD, and ulcerative colitis[21]
- Ameliorates rheumatoid inflammation[21]
- **Attenuated high fat diet induced nonalcoholic fatty liver disease in mice**[22]
- **Corrected high fat diet induced gut microbiota imbalance**[22]
- **Elevated abundances of beneficial bacteria**[22]
- **Restored high fat diet induced intestinal mucosa damage**[22]
- Increased expression of ZO-1 in small intestine[22]
- Decreased the levels of gut endotoxin in serum and liver compared with high fat group[22]
- Downregulated endotoxin associated genes TLR4 and Myd88 and pro-inflammation genes such as MCP-1, TNF-α, IL-1, IL-2, IL-6 and IFN-γ in liver or epididymal fat[22]
- **Ameliorated liver inflammation and fat accumulation**[22]
- **Reduced triglyceride and cholesterol levels in liver**[22]
- NAS score was decreased[22]
- FBG and HOMA-IR and ALT and AST were improved[22]
- Stimulates appetite suppressing hormones[23]
- Increases capacity for cold induced thermogenesis[23]
- Completely blocked high fat diet induced weight gain in mice[23]
- Reduced fasting insulin and leptin levels[23]
- Protects against diet-induced obesity in mice[23]
- At low concentration promotes intestinal barrier function as measured by transepithelial electrical resistance[24]
- At high concentration reduces TER and increases gut permeability[24]
- Increases colonic blood flow[25]
- May enhance colonic anastomosis healing[25]
- May reduce the symptoms of ulcerative colitis and may prevent the progression of colitis in general[25]
- Regulates GPR41-mediated sympathetic nervous system activity controlling body energy expenditure and maintaining metabolic homeostasis[13]
- Increases expression of trefoil factors (TFFs), which are mucin-associated peptides that help maintain and repair the intestinal mucosa[13]
- Stimulates the production of antimicrobial peptides such as IL-37[13]
- Decreases IBS symptoms[26]
- Increases the effectiveness of peristalsis[26]
- Counteracts acute dehydration from diarrhoea[26]

- Decreases symptoms of diverticulosis[26]
- Upregulates the expression of tight junction proteins[4]
- Enhances intestinal barrier by regulating the assembly of tight junctions[5]
- Promotes reassembly of tight-junctions[6]
- Represses permeability-promoting claudin-2 tight-junction protein expression[7]
- Enhances mRNA expression of the intestinal mucosal tight junction proteins occludin and zonula occluden protein-1[8]

References:
1.Rivière A, Selak M, Lantin D, Leroy F, De Vuyst L. Bifidobacteria and Butyrate-Producing Colon Bacteria: Importance and Strategies for Their Stimulation in the Human Gut. Front Microbiol. 2016;7:979. Published 2016 Jun 28. doi:10.3389/fmicb.2016.00979

2. Canani RB, Costanzo MD, Leone L, Pedata M, Meli R, Calignano A. Potential beneficial effects of butyrate in intestinal and extraintestinal diseases. World J Gastroenterol. 2011;17(12):1519-28.

3. Cushing K, Alvarado DM, Ciorba MA. Butyrate and Mucosal Inflammation: New Scientific Evidence Supports Clinical Observation. Clin Transl Gastroenterol. 2015;6(8):e108. Published 2015 Aug 27. doi:10.1038/ctg.2015.34

4. Yan, Hui, and Kolapo M Ajuwon. "Butyrate modifies intestinal barrier function in IPEC-J2 cells through a selective upregulation of tight junction proteins and activation of the Akt signaling pathway." PloS one vol. 12,6 e0179586. 27 Jun. 2017, doi:10.1371/journal.pone.0179586

5. Peng, Luying et al. "Butyrate enhances the intestinal barrier by facilitating tight junction assembly via activation of AMP-activated protein kinase in Caco-2 cell monolayers." The Journal of nutrition vol. 139,9 (2009): 1619-25. doi:10.3945/jn.109.104638

6. Miao, Wei et al. "Sodium Butyrate Promotes Reassembly of Tight Junctions in Caco-2 Monolayers Involving Inhibition of MLCK/MLC2 Pathway and Phosphorylation of PKCβ2." International journal of molecular sciences vol. 17,10 1696. 10 Oct. 2016, doi:10.3390/ijms17101696

7. Zheng, Leon et al. "Microbial-Derived Butyrate Promotes Epithelial Barrier Function through IL-10 Receptor-Dependent Repression of Claudin-2." Journal of immunology (Baltimore, Md. : 1950) vol. 199,8 (2017): 2976-2984. doi:10.4049/jimmunol.1700105

8. Ma X, Fan PX, Li LS, Qiao SY, Zhang GL, Li DF. Butyrate promotes the recovering of intestinal wound healing through its positive effect on the tight junctions. J Anim Sci. 2012 Dec;90 Suppl 4:266-8. doi: 10.2527/jas.50965. PMID: 23365351.

9. Ríos-Covián D, Ruas-Madiedo P, Margolles A, Gueimonde M, de Los Reyes-Gavilán CG, Salazar N. Intestinal Short Chain Fatty Acids and their Link with Diet and Human Health. Front Microbiol. 2016;7:185. Published 2016 Feb 17. doi:10.3389/fmicb.2016.00185

10. Puddu A, Sanguineti R, Montecucco F, Viviani GL. Evidence for the gut microbiota short-chain fatty acids as key pathophysiological molecules improving diabetes. Mediators Inflamm. 2014;2014:162021.

11. den Besten G, van Eunen K, Groen AK, Venema K, Reijngoud DJ, Bakker BM. The role of short-chain fatty acids in the interplay between diet, gut microbiota, and host energy metabolism. J Lipid Res. 2013;54(9):2325-40.

12. Wong JM, de Souza R, Kendall CW, Emam A, Jenkins DJ. Colonic health: fermentation and short chain fatty acids. *J Clin Gastroenterol.* 2006 Mar;40(3):235-43. doi: 10.1097/00004836-200603000-00015. PMID: 16633129.

13. Liu, Hu et al. "Butyrate: A Double-Edged Sword for Health?." *Advances in nutrition (Bethesda, Md.)* vol. 9,1 (2018): 21-29. doi:10.1093/advances/nmx009

14. Vital, Marius et al. "Colonic Butyrate-Producing Communities in Humans: an Overview Using

Omics Data." *mSystems* vol. 2,6 e00130-17. 5 Dec. 2017, doi:10.1128/mSystems.00130-17

15. Sossai P. Butyric acid: what is the future for this old substance? Swiss Med Wkly. 2012 Jun 6;142:w13596. doi: 10.4414/smw.2012.13596. PMID: 22674349.

16. Li Z, Yi C, Katiraei S, et alButyrate reduces appetite and activates brown adipose tissue via the gut-brain neural circuitGut 2018;67:1269-1279.

17. Donohoe DR, Garge N, Zhang X, et al. The microbiome and butyrate regulate energy metabolism and autophagy in the mammalian colon. Cell Metab. 2011;13(5):517-26.

18. Meijer K, de Vos P, Priebe MG. Butyrate and other short-chain fatty acids as modulators of immunity: what relevance for health? Curr Opin Clin Nutr Metab Care. 2010 Nov;13(6):715-21. doi: 10.1097/MCO.0b013e32833eebe5. PMID: 20823773.

19. Matt, Stephanie M et al. "Butyrate and Dietary Soluble Fiber Improve Neuroinflammation Associated With Aging in Mice." Frontiers in immunology vol. 9 1832. 14 Aug. 2018, doi:10.3389/fimmu.2018.01832

20. Schwarz A, Bruhs A, Schwarz T. The Short-Chain Fatty Acid Sodium Butyrate Functions as a Regulator of the Skin Immune System. J Invest Dermatol. 2017 Apr;137(4):855-864. doi: 10.1016/j.jid.2016.11.014. Epub 2016 Nov 23. PMID: 27887954.

21. Kim DS, Kwon JE, Lee SH, et al. Attenuation of Rheumatoid Inflammation by Sodium Butyrate Through Reciprocal Targeting of HDAC2 in Osteoclasts and HDAC8 in T Cells. Front Immunol. 2018;9:1525. Published 2018 Jul 6. doi:10.3389/fimmu.2018.01525

22. Zhou D, Pan Q, Xin FZ, et al. Sodium butyrate attenuates high-fat diet-induced steatohepatitis in mice by improving gut microbiota and gastrointestinal barrier. World J Gastroenterol. 2017;23(1):60-75.

23. Lin HV, Frassetto A, Kowalik EJ, et al. Butyrate and propionate protect against diet-induced obesity and regulate gut hormones via free fatty acid receptor 3-independent mechanisms. PLoS One. 2012;7(4):e35240.

24. Peng L, He Z, Chen W, Holzman IR, Lin J. Effects of butyrate on intestinal barrier function in a Caco-2 cell monolayer model of intestinal barrier. Pediatr Res. 2007 Jan;61(1):37-41. doi: 10.1203/01.pdr.0000250014.92242.f3. PMID: 17211138.

25. Velázquez OC, Lederer HM, Rombeau JL. Butyrate and the colonocyte. Production, absorption, metabolism, and therapeutic implications. Adv Exp Med Biol. 1997;427:123-34. PMID: 9361838.

26. Borycka-Kiciak, Katarzyna et al. "Butyric acid - a well-known molecule revisited." Przeglad gastroenterologiczny vol. 12,2 (2017): 83-89. doi:10.5114/pg.2017.68342

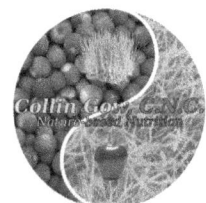

Resources

Vaccine Information Resources

Documentaries

1. The Silent Epidemic: The Untold Story of Vaccines (2013) (Gary Null, Ph.D.)
2. Vaccine Nation (2008) (Gary Null, Ph.D.)
3. The Quiet Killer - The Exploding Autoimmune Epidemics – Vaccines and Man Made Cancer – Dr. Randy Tent (Dr. Randy Tent)
4. Death By Medicine (2011) (Gary Null, Ph.D.)
5. Shots in the Dark: Silence on Vaccine (2009) (Lina B. Moreco)
6. Vaxxed: From Cover-up to Catastrophe (2016) (Dr. Andrew Wakefield)
7. Vaccination: The Hidden Truth (1998)
8. Hear the Silence (2003) (Dr. Andrew Wakefield)
9. Autism: Made in the USA (2009) (Gary Null, Ph.D.)
10. Deadly Deception (Gary Null Ph.D.)
11. In Lies We Trust – The CIA, Hollywood, and Bioterrorism (Leonard G. Horowitz)

Books

1. Miller's Review of Critical Vaccine Studies: 400 Important Scientific Papers Summarized for Parents and Researchers (2016) (Neil Z. Miller)
2. Dr. Mary's Monkey (2015) (Edward T. Haslam)
3. Thimerosal: Let the Science Speak: The Evidence Supporting the Immediate Removal of Mercury–a Known Neurotoxin–from Vaccines (2014) (Robert F. Kennedy Jr.)
4. Death By Medicine (2010) (Gary Null, Ph.D.)
5. Emerging Viruses – AIDS and Ebola (1996) (Leonard G. Horowitz)

Vaccine Ingredients

https://www.cdc.gov/vaccines/pubs/pinkbook/downloads/appendices/b/excipient-table-2.pdf

Summary-Excipients Included in U.S. Vaccines by Vaccine-February 2020   1 / 4

Vaccine Excipient Summary
Excipients Included in U.S. Vaccines, by Vaccine

In addition to weakened or killed disease antigens (viruses or bacteria), vaccines contain very small amounts of other ingredients – excipients.

Some excipients are added to a vaccine for a specific purpose. These include:
Preservatives, to prevent contamination. For example, thimerosal.
Adjuvants, to help stimulate a stronger immune response. For example, aluminum salts.
Stabilizers, to keep the vaccine potent during transportation and storage. For example, sugars or gelatin.

Others are residual trace amounts of materials that were used during the manufacturing process and removed. These can include:
Cell culture materials, used to grow the vaccine antigens. For example, egg protein, various culture media.
Inactivating ingredients, used to kill viruses or inactivate toxins. For example, formaldehyde.
Antibiotics, used to prevent contamination by bacteria. For example, neomycin.

The following table lists substances, other than active ingredients (i.e., antigens), shown in the manufacturers' package insert (PI) as being contained in the final formulation of each vaccine. **Note: Substances used in the manufacture of a vaccine but not listed as contained in the final product (e.g., culture media) can be found in each PI, but are not shown on this table.** Each PI, which can be found on the FDA's website (see below) contains a description of that vaccine's manufacturing process, including the amount and purpose of each substance. In most PIs, this information is found in Section 11: "Description."

All information was extracted from manufacturers' package inserts.
The date shown in the Date column of the table is the edition date of the PI is use in February 2020.
If a date contains an asterisk (*), the PI was not dated and this is the date the PI was reviewed for this table.
If in doubt about whether a PI has been updated since this table was prepared, check the FDA's website at:
http://www.fda.gov/BiologicsBloodVaccines/Vaccines/ApprovedProducts/ucm093833.htm
All influenza vaccine in this table are 2019-20 northern hemisphere formulation.

Vaccine	Date	Contains
Adenovirus	10/2019	monosodium glutamate, sucrose, D-mannose, D-fructose, dextrose, human serum albumin, potassium phosphate, plasdone C, anhydrous lactose, microcrystalline

Available for download @ collingowcnc.wixsite.com/collingowcnc/articlesandprotocols

These statements have not been evaluated by the FDA. This is not an attempt to treat, diagnose, prevent, or cure any disease or condition. Talk to your doctor before making any changes.

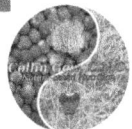

Gut Problems?

Leaky gut? IBS? IBD? UC? Diverticulosis? Constipation?
Food Sensitivities? Autoimmunity? Overweight?

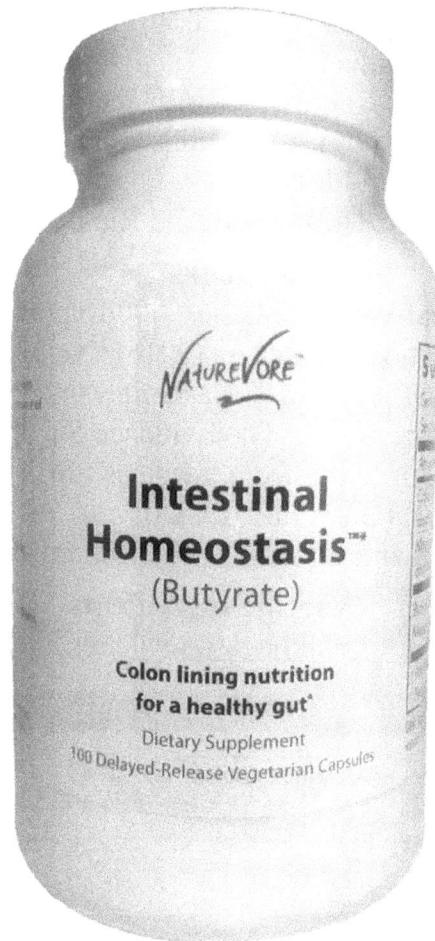

* **Powerful** *
Postbiotic!

* **Fuel For** *
Colon Cells!

NATUREVORE

Intestinal Homeostasis™
(Butyrate)

Colon lining nutrition
for a healthy gut*
Dietary Supplement
100 Delayed-Release Vegetarian Capsules

Over 40 clinically proven
beneficial effects of butyrate can't be wrong!

↑Tight Junctions* ↑Gut Barrier Integrity* ↓Inflammation*
↑Beneficial Bacteria* ↑Absorption* ↓Appetite* •Antioxidant*
•Antitumor* •Modulates G.I. Motility* & Innate Immunity*
•Supports Normal Intestinal PH* & Intestinal Mucosa Homeostasis*
↓Insulin Resistance* ↑Metabolism* ↑Antimicrobial Peptides*
•Modulates Neuronal Excitability* ↑Glutathione* ↓Endotoxins*

For References and to Purchase: collingowcnc.wixsite.com/collingowcnc/intestinalhomeostasis

*These statements have not been evaluated by the FDA. This product is not intended to treat, diagnose, prevent, or cure any disease or condition.

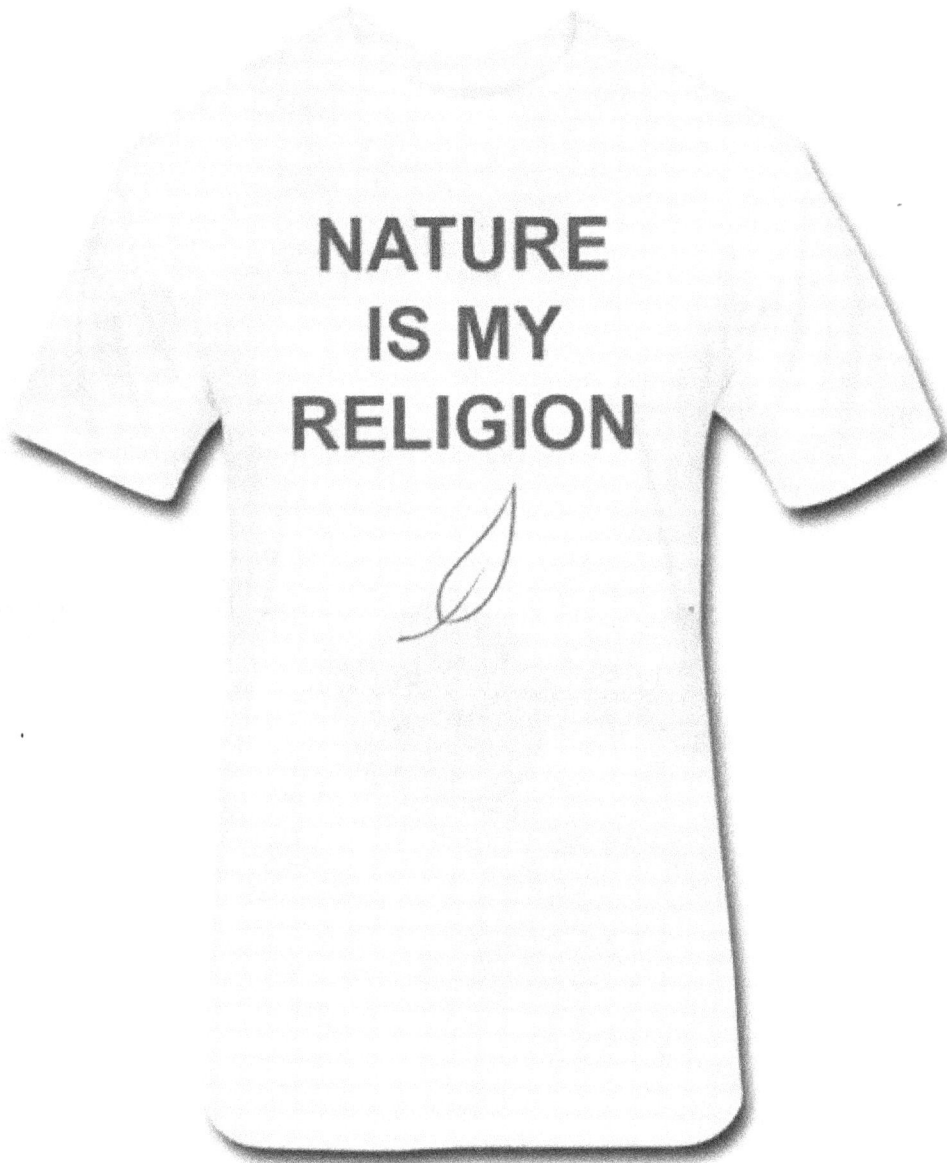

NATURE
IS MY
RELIGION

Buy Here: https://collingowcnc.wixsite.com/collingowcnc/t-shirts

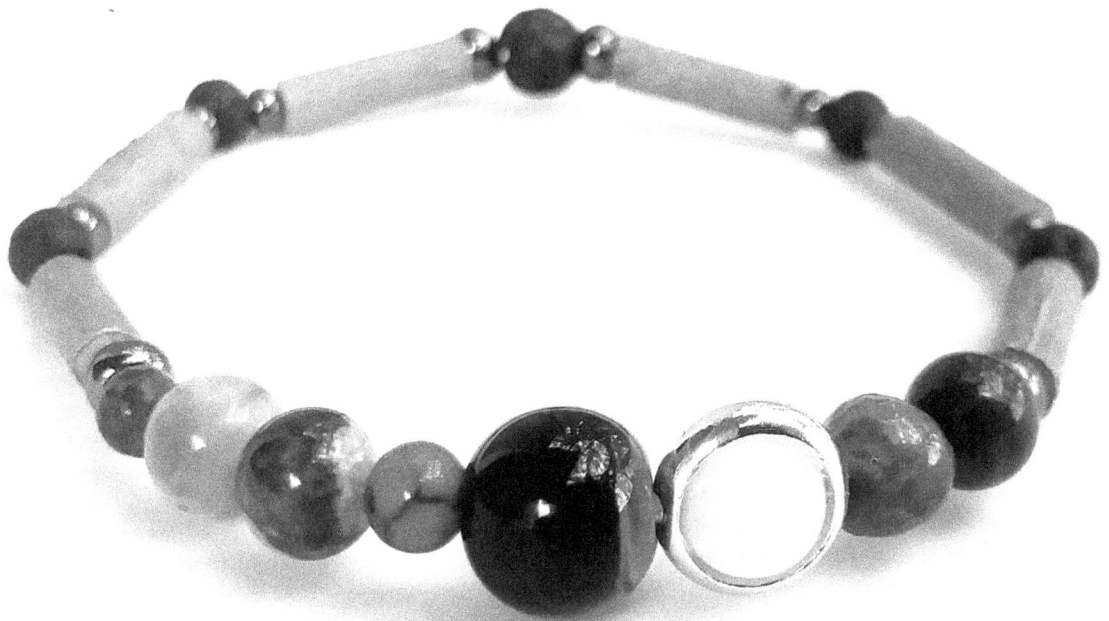

Fullscript

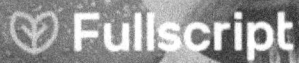

The safest source for practitioner-grade supplements.

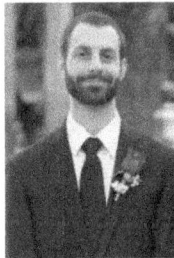

Email *

Submit

Supplement Store: https://us.fullscript.com/welcome/collingowcnc

https://collingowcnc.wixsite.com/collingowcnc

Collin Gow, C.N.C.

Nature-based Nutrition, Diet, and Lifestyle

Español Français Русский

Follow Us

Home   About   Shop   Health & Nutrition Videos   Articles & Protocols   Book A Consultation   Contact

Shop

BOOKS

INTESTINAL HOMEOSTASIS
Homeostasis
(Butyrate)

NATURE
IS MY
T-SHIRTS

BRACELETS

SUPPLEMENT STORE

Slideshow

Instagram Feed

powers amid coronavirus
pandemic

Corona

False Information Found on Collin Gow, CNC

Collin Gow CNC posted information that's been reviewed by Lead Stories. We've added a notice to the post so others can see that it's false.

Collin Gow, C.N.C.

is a certified nutritional consultant, health expert, author, artist, entrepreneur, naturevore, naturotheologist, lover of nature, astrology, numerology, astrotheology, ethnography, and much more!

Collin's Websites

www.collingowcnc.wixsite.com/collingowcnc
www.collingowcnc.com (under construction as of 12/31/2020)
www.collingowcnc.wixsite.com/naturevorenutrition
www.naturevorenutrition.com (under construction as of 12/31/2020)
www.collingowcnc.wixsite.com/naturotheology
www.naturotheology.org (under construction as of 12/31/2020)

Collin's Other Books

The Night Before Winter Solstice:
An Earth and Nature-Based Spin on a Christmas Classic
Available for purchase on Amazon @
https://www.amazon.com/Night-Before-Winter-Solstice-Nature-Based/dp/0578828634/ref=sr_1_2?
dchild=1&keywords=the+night+before+winter+solstice&qid=1609474209&sr=8-2

www.ingramcontent.com/pod-product-compliance
Lightning Source LLC
Chambersburg PA
CBHW080617270326
41928CB00016B/3102